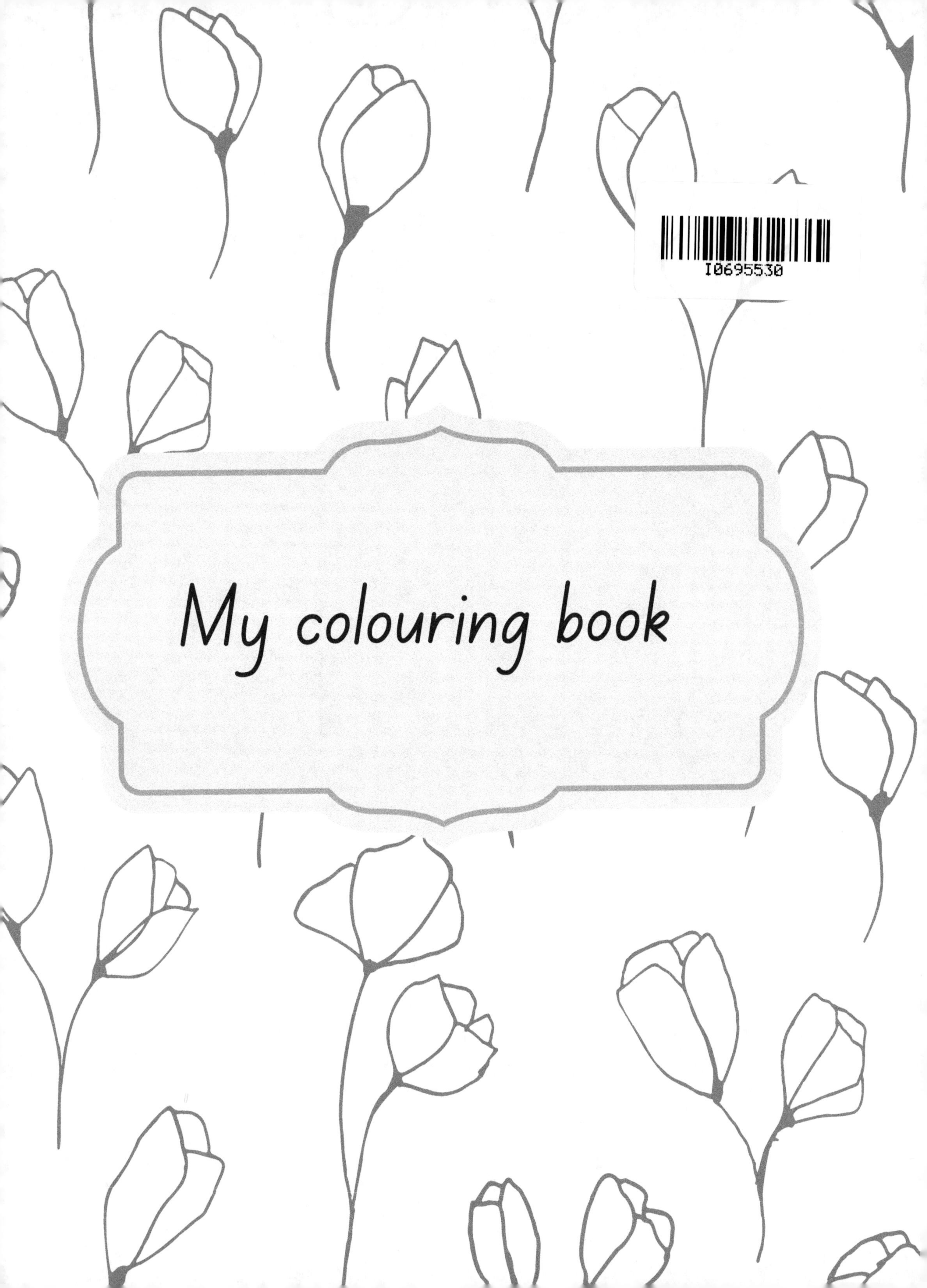

My colouring book

Jasmine

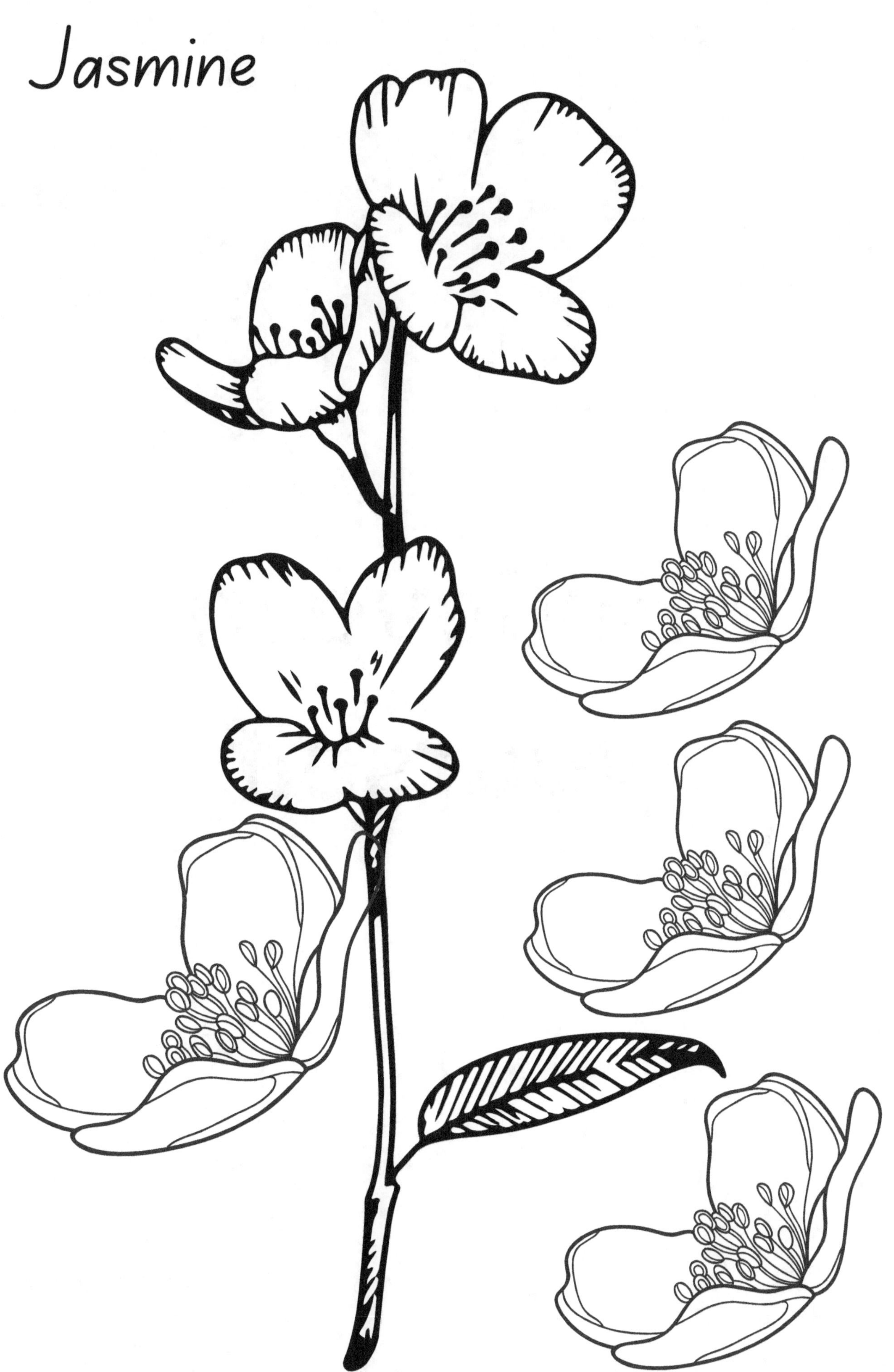

Believe in yourself

Bougainvillea

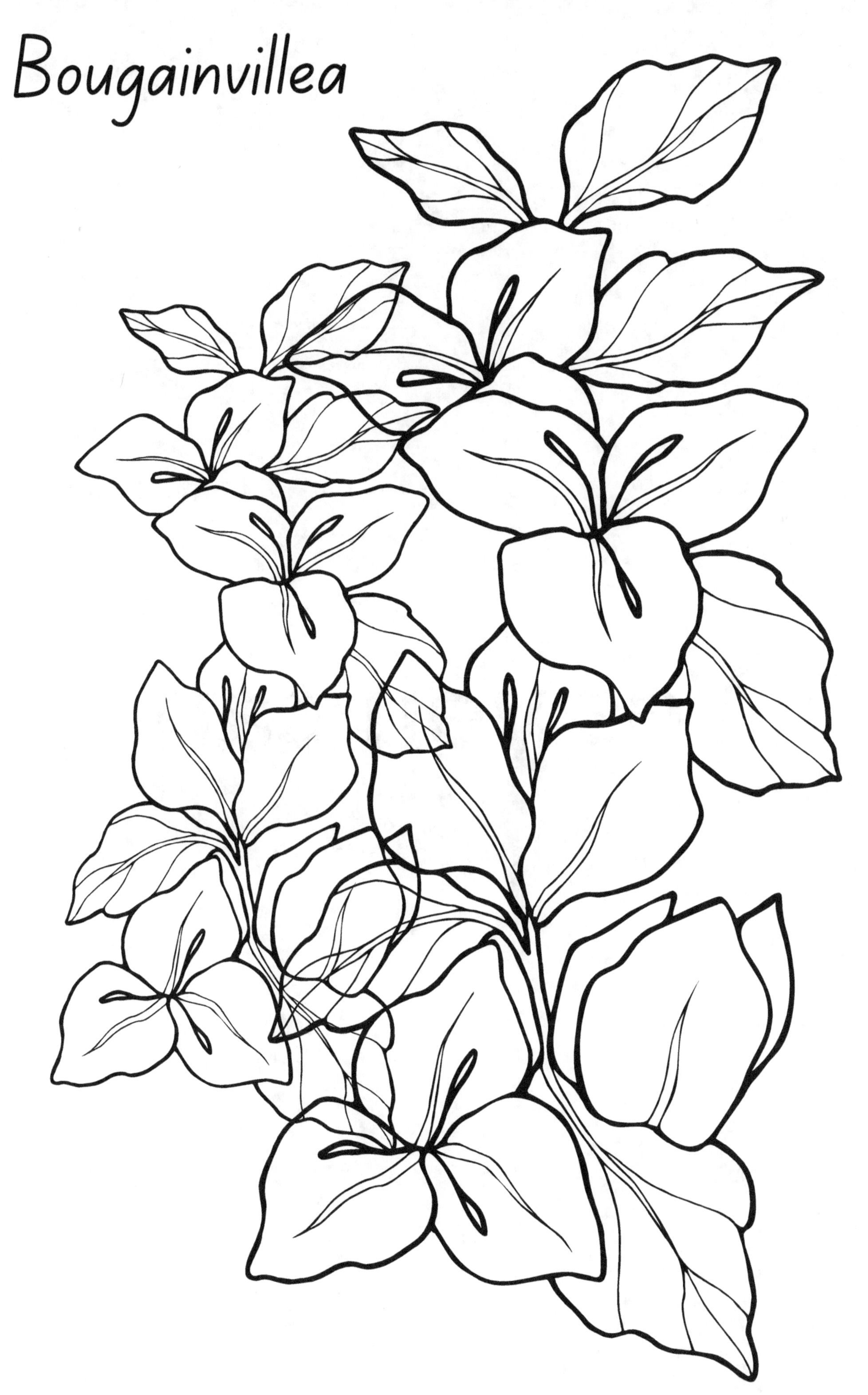

Yes you can

Chrysanthemum

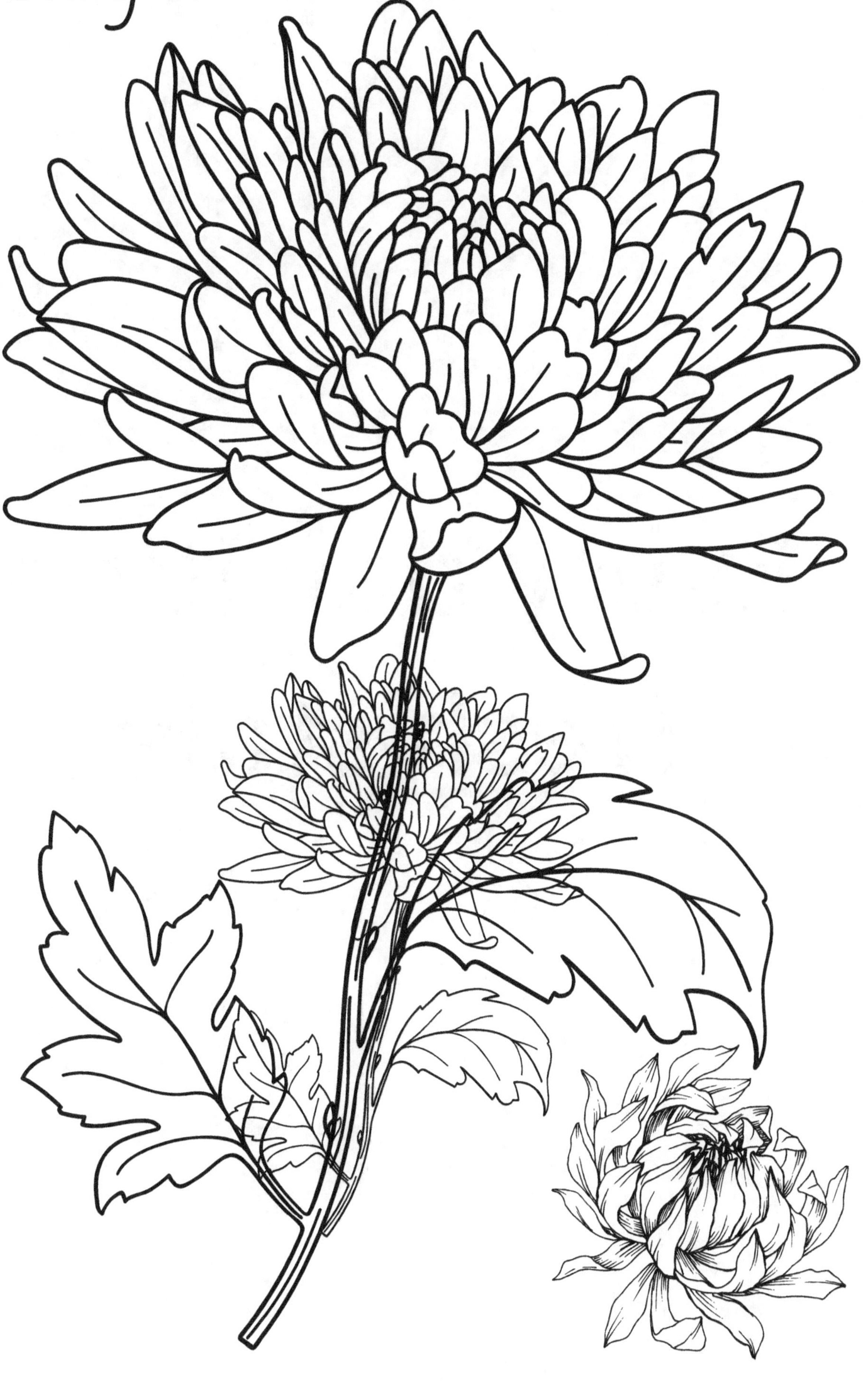

Every day it's a fresh start

Tuberose

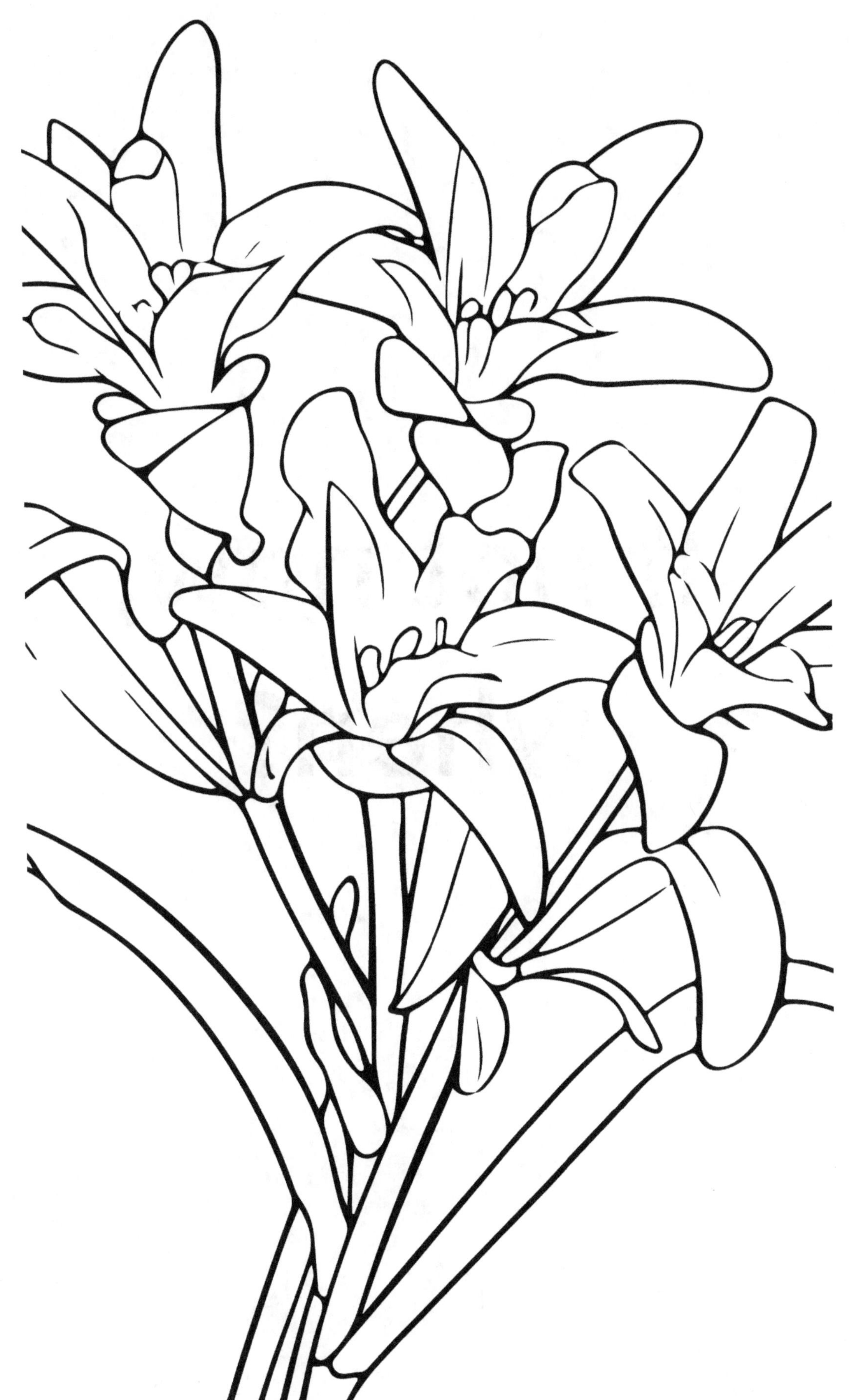

If not now, when?

Daffodil

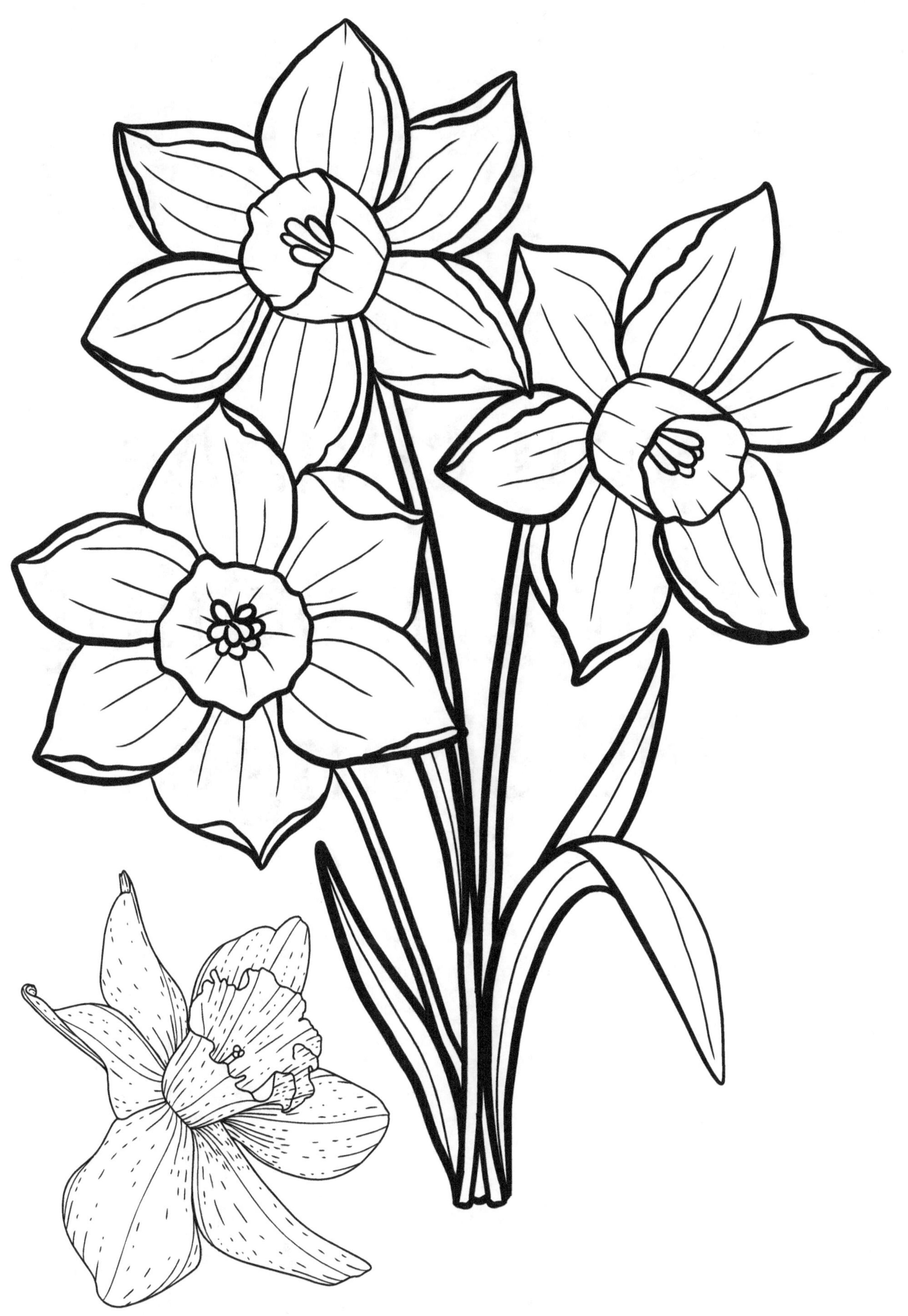

If you change nothing, nothing will change

Snowdrop

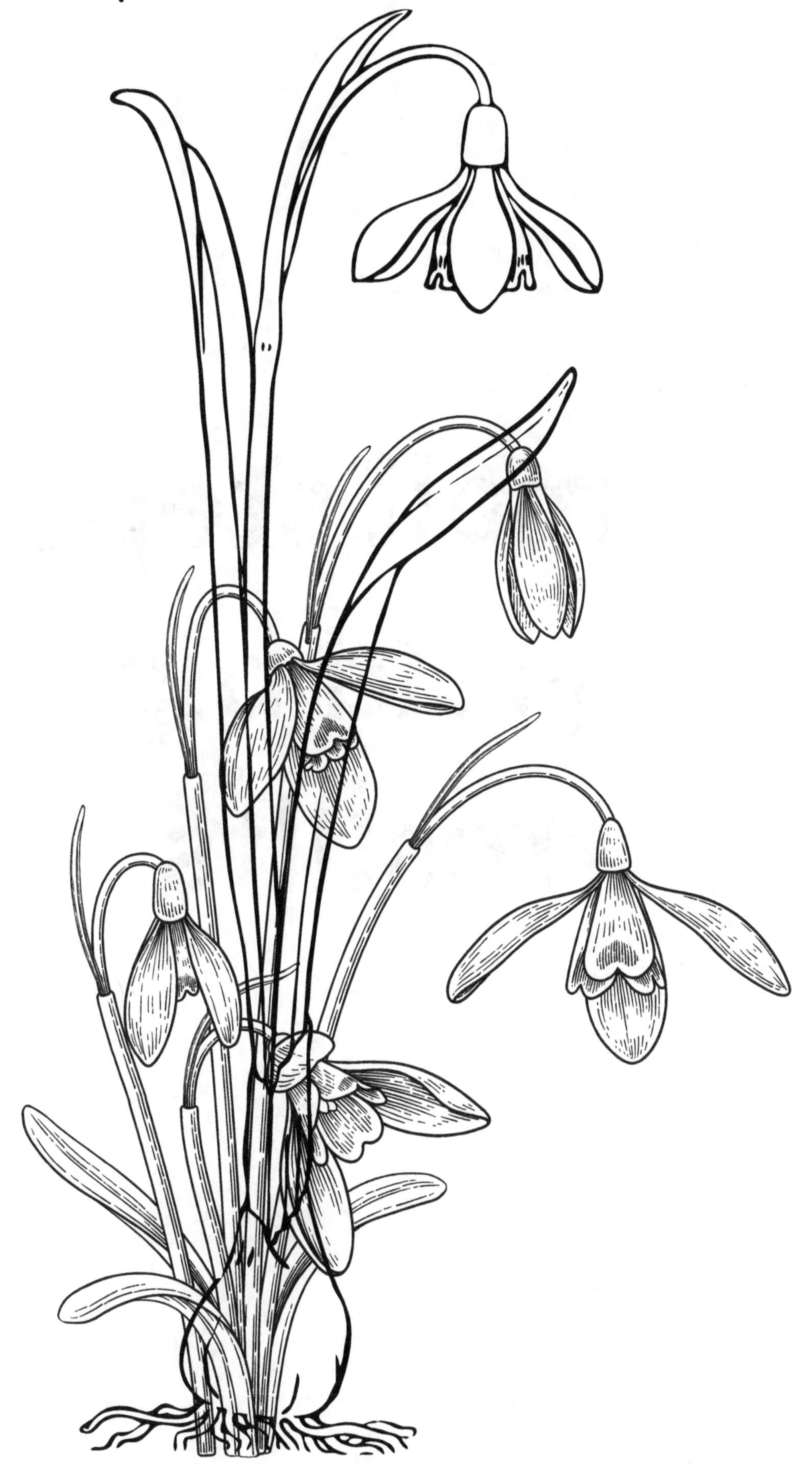

Small steps yield big results

Sunflower

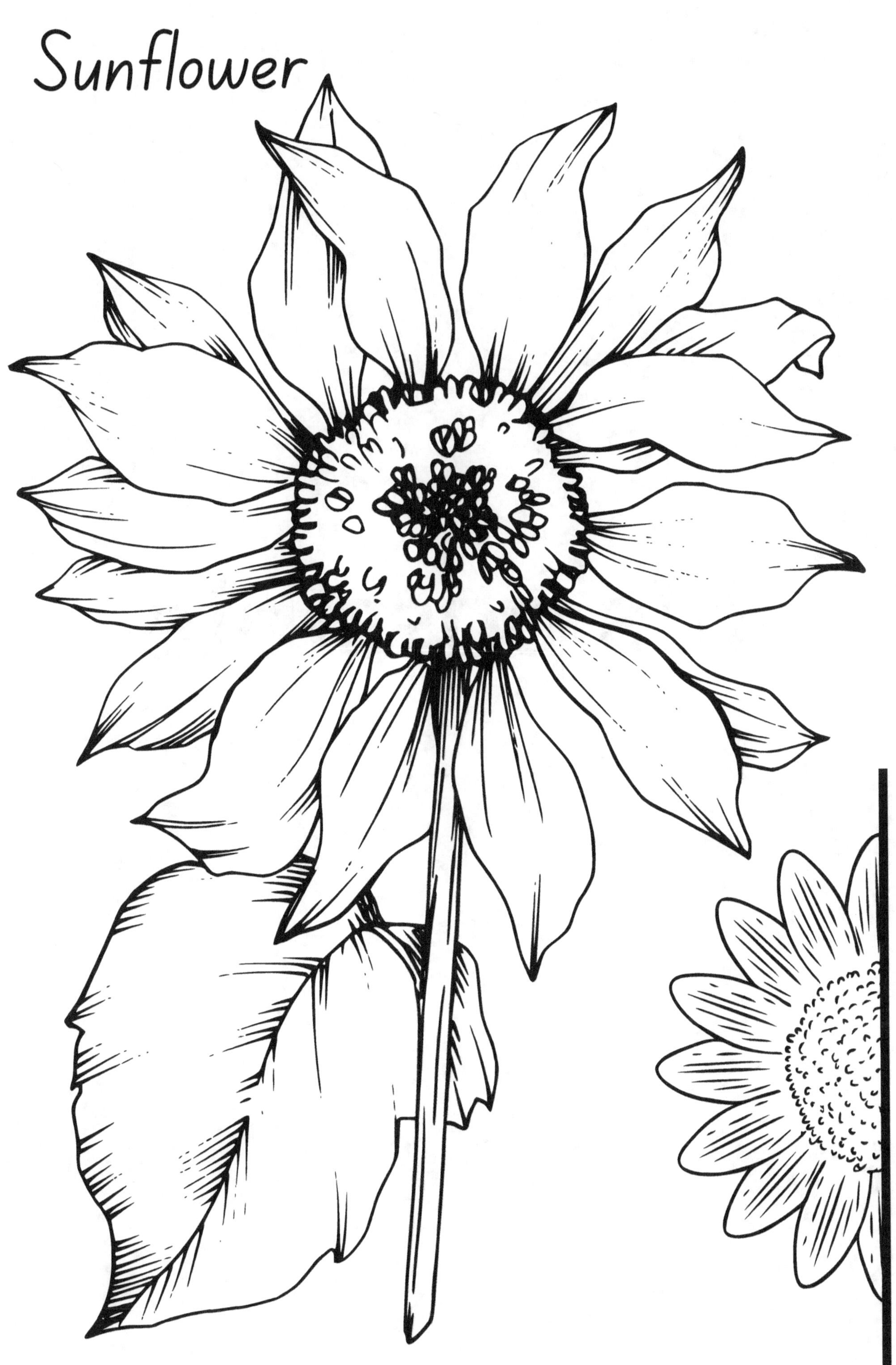

It's possible

Hyacinth

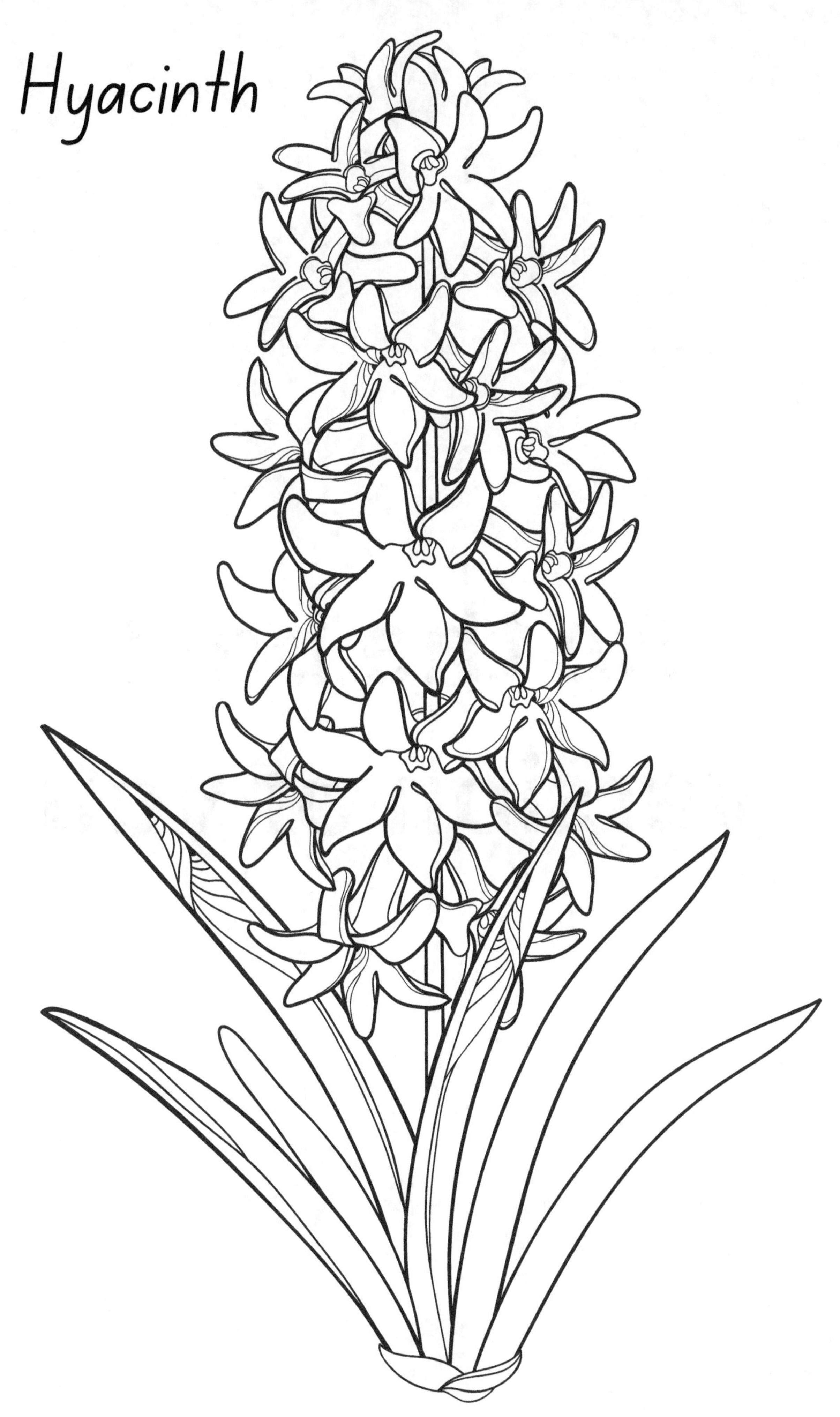

Be the best version of you

Carnation

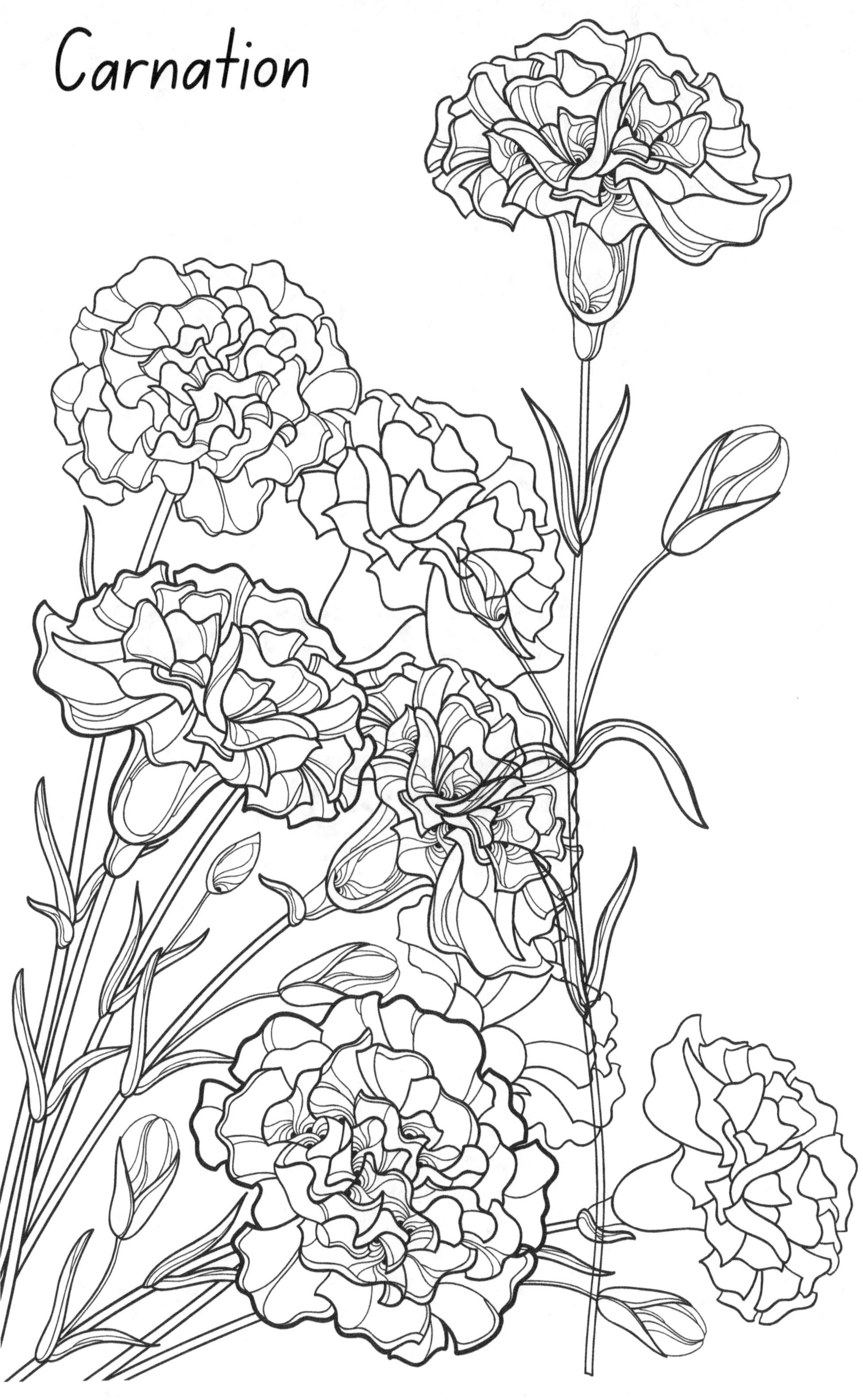

Inspire someone today

Lotus

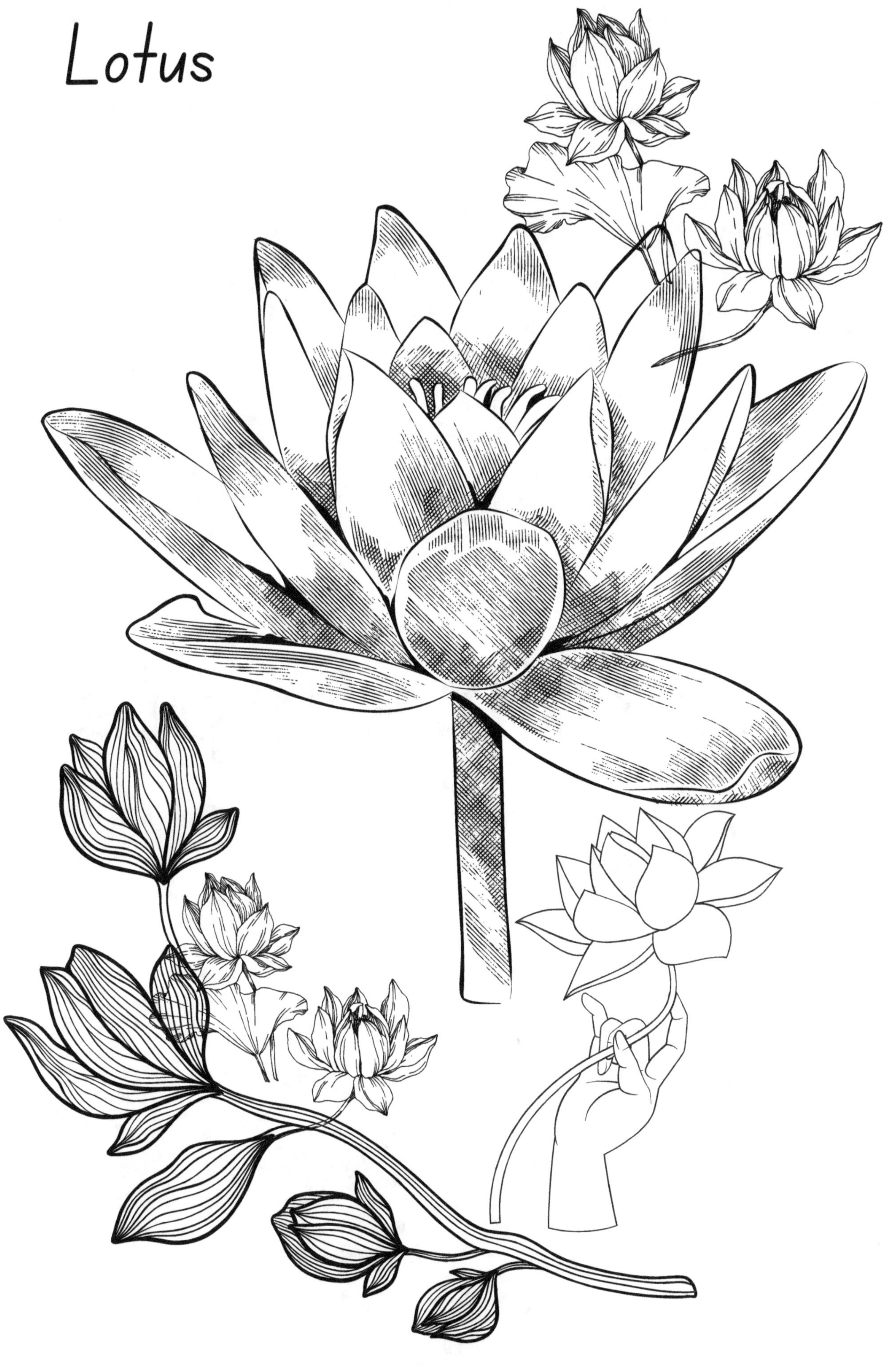

Keep it simple

Marigold

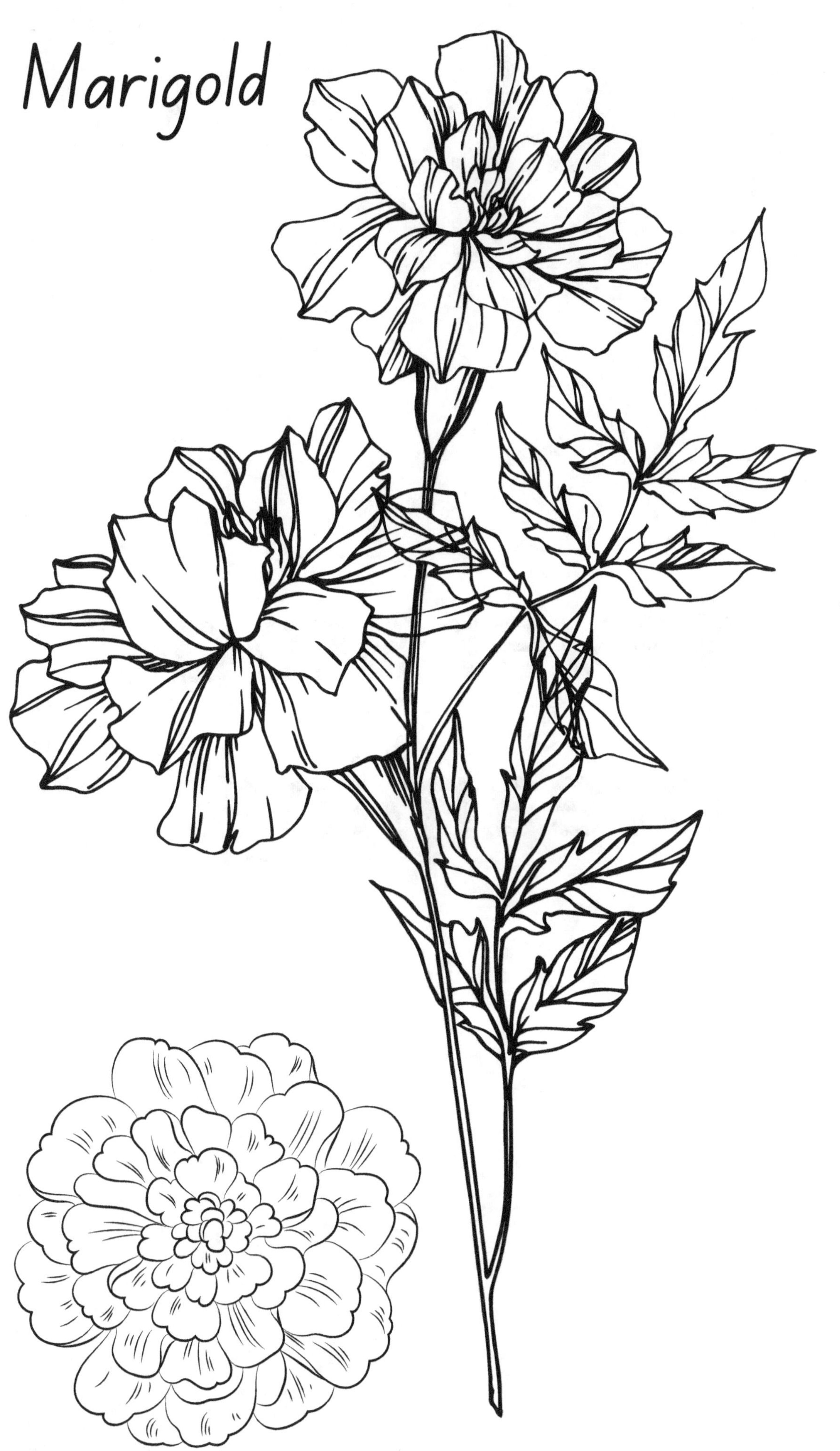

Never stop dreaming

Gladiolus

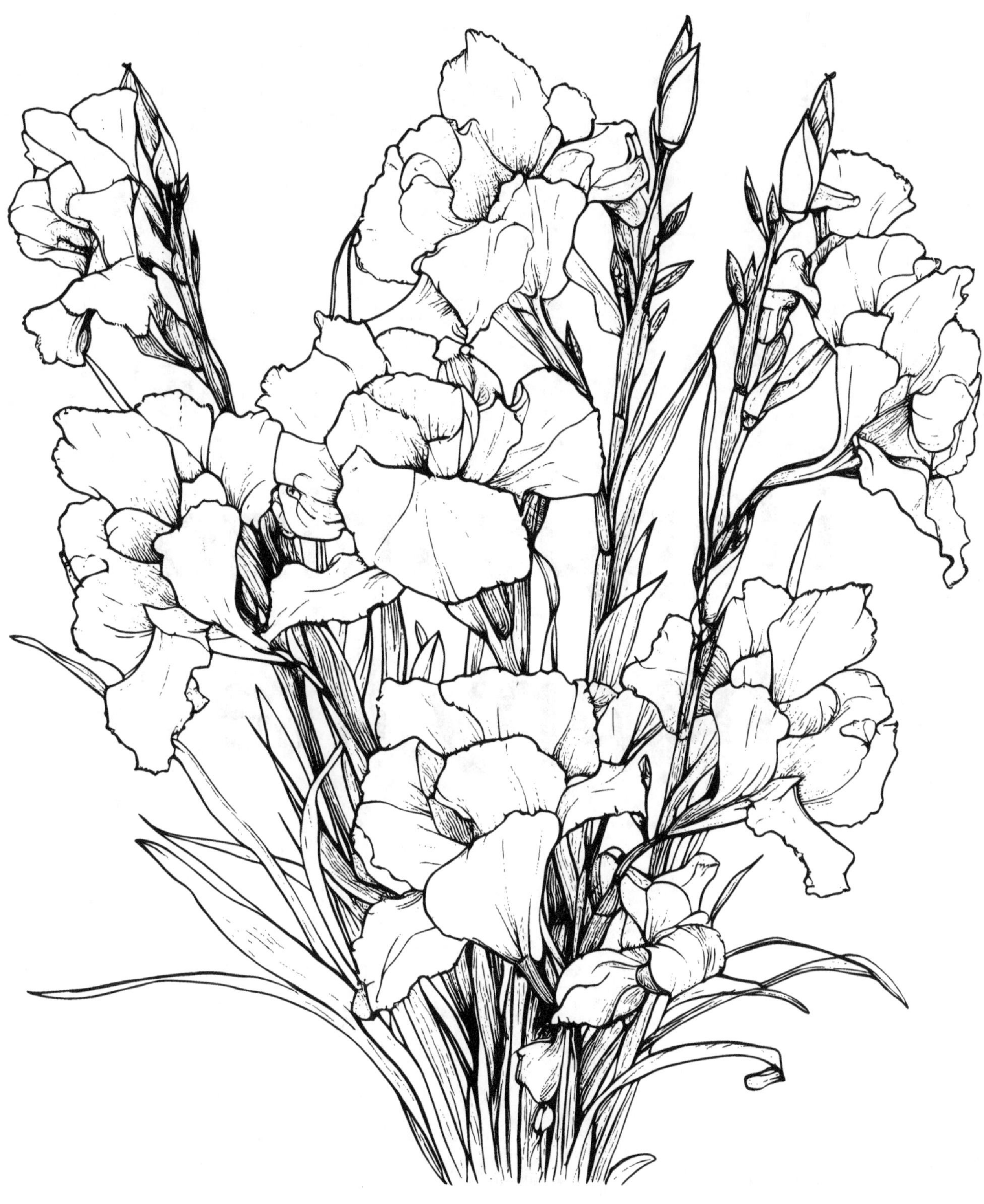

Happy mind
happy life

Orchid

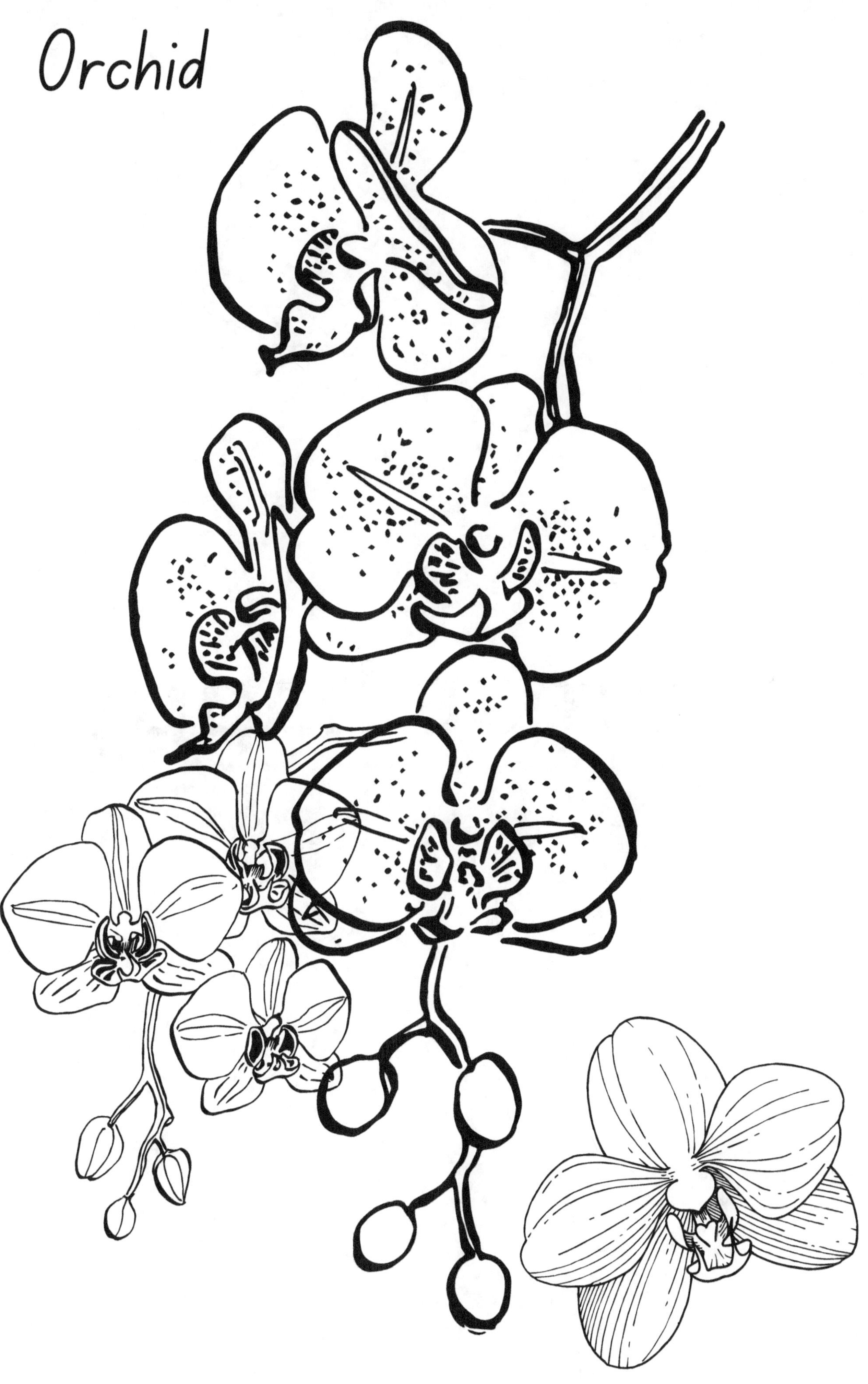

Choose happy

Lily

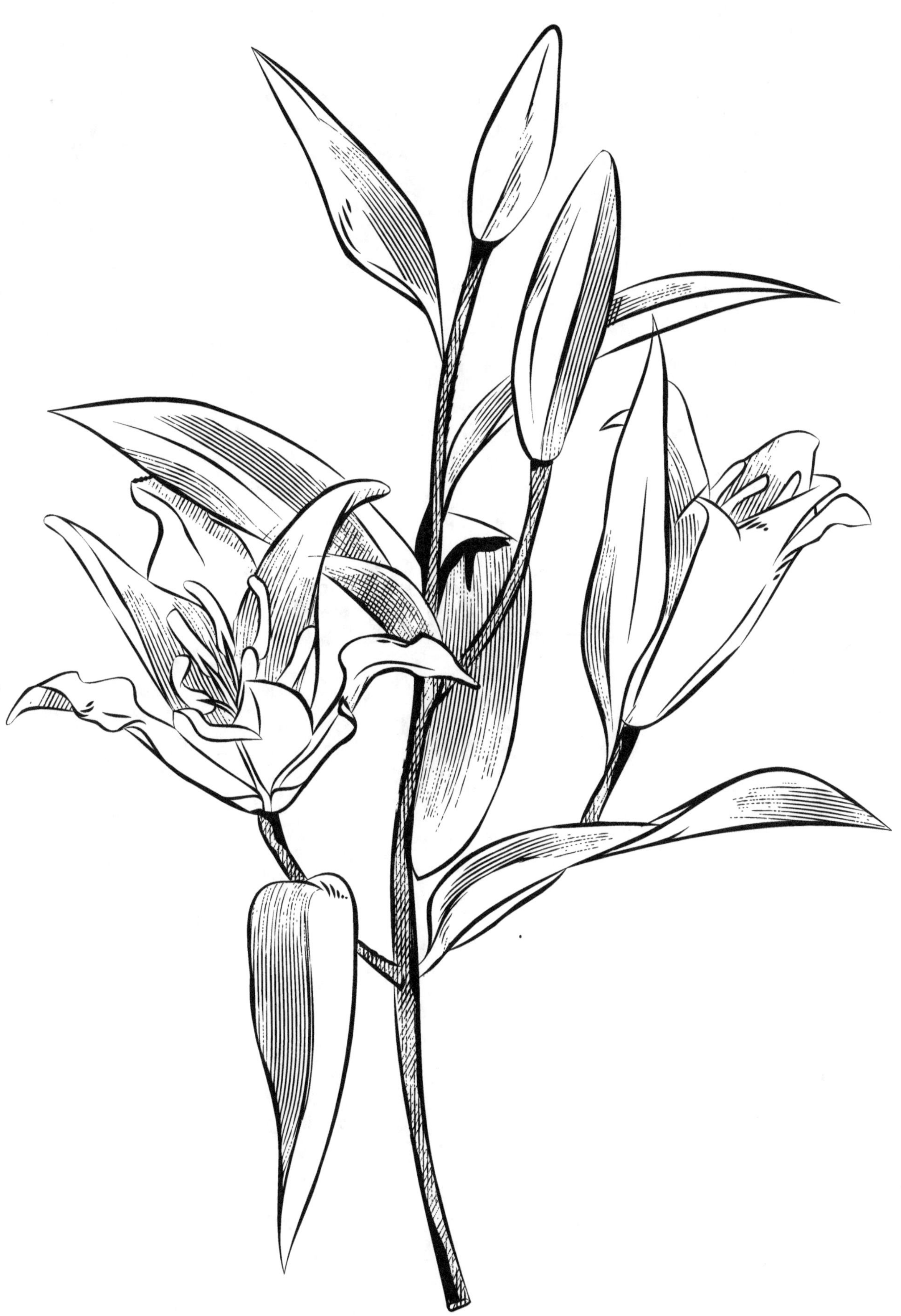

Smile

Lily of the valley

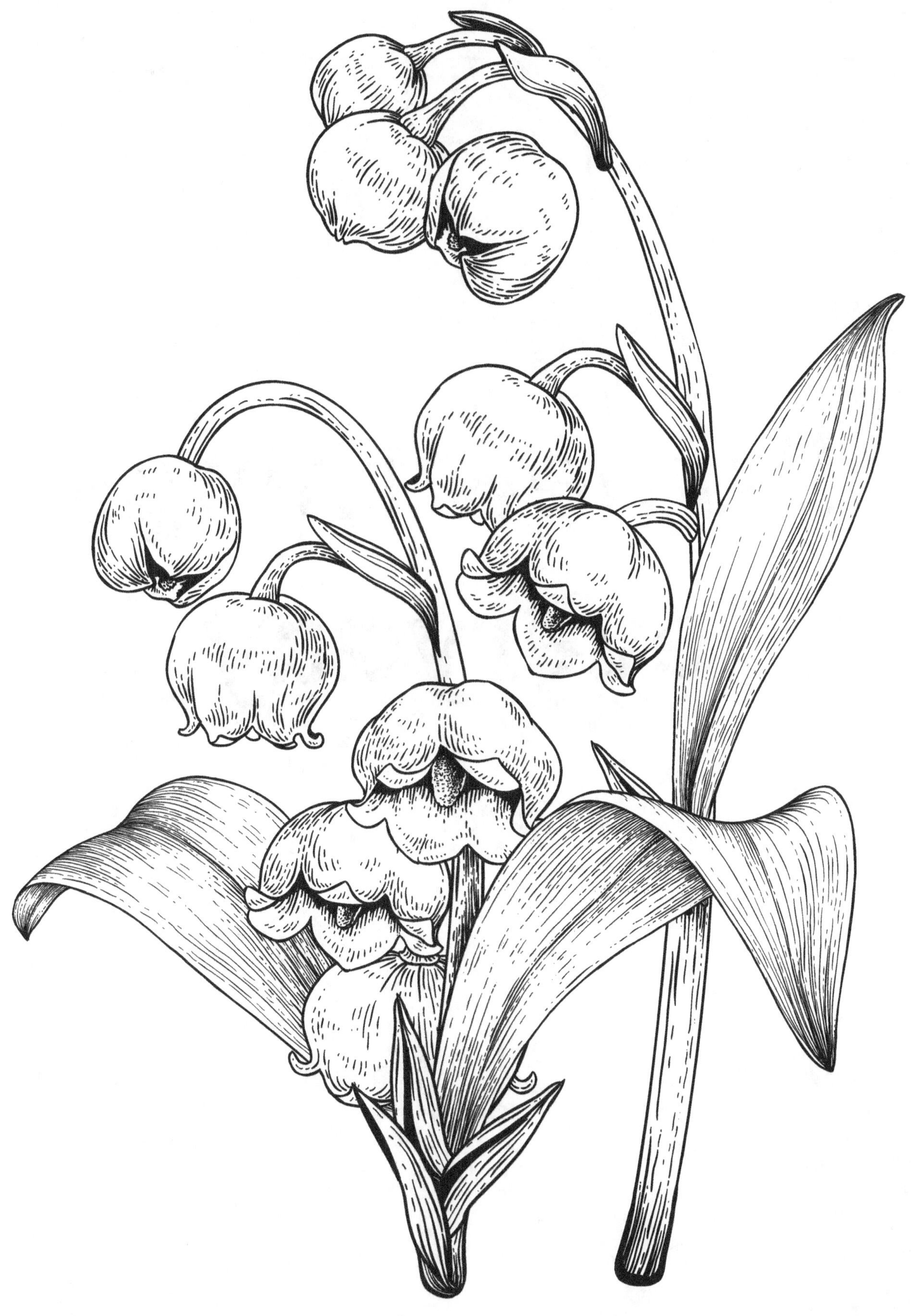

Do new things
everyday

Poppy

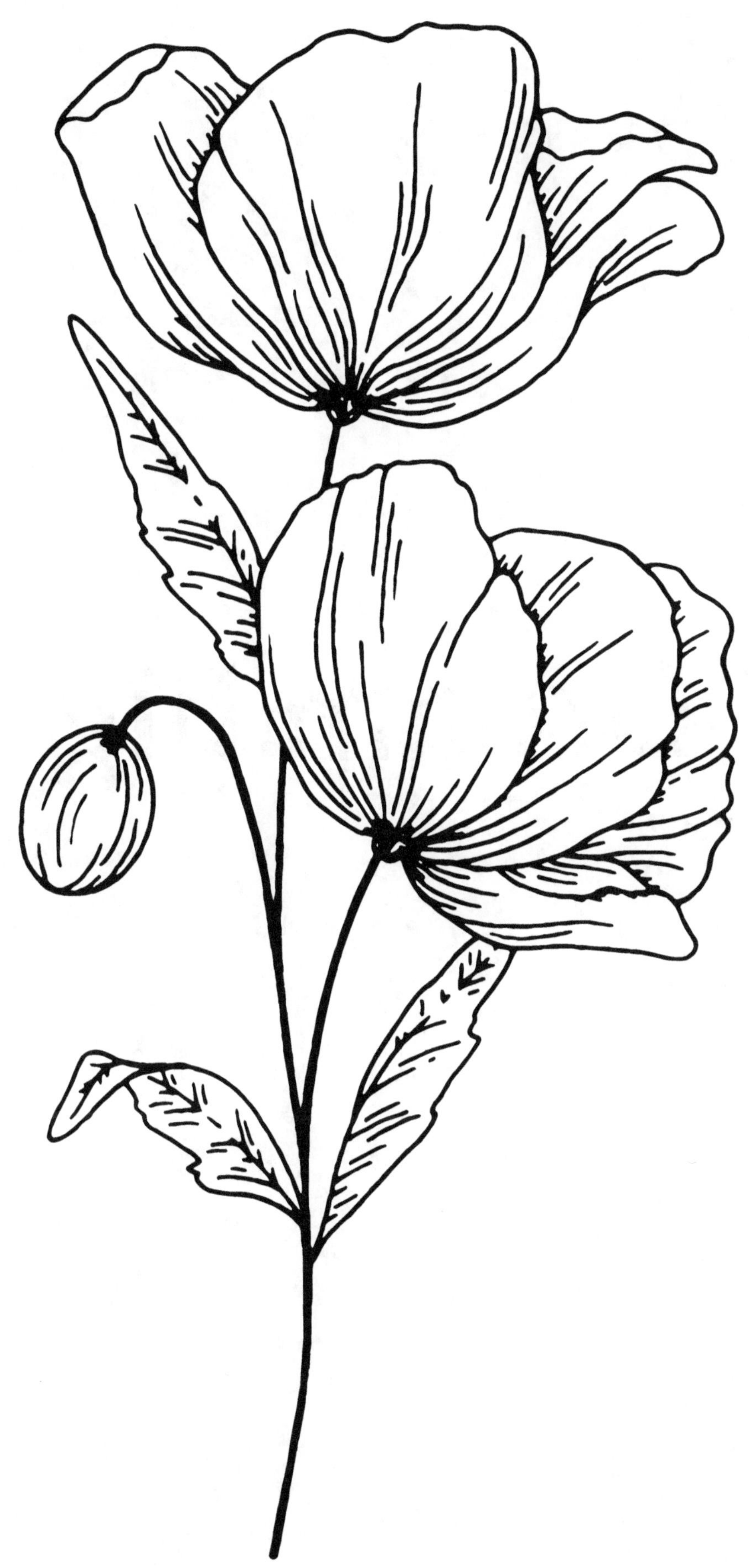

Dream big

Peony

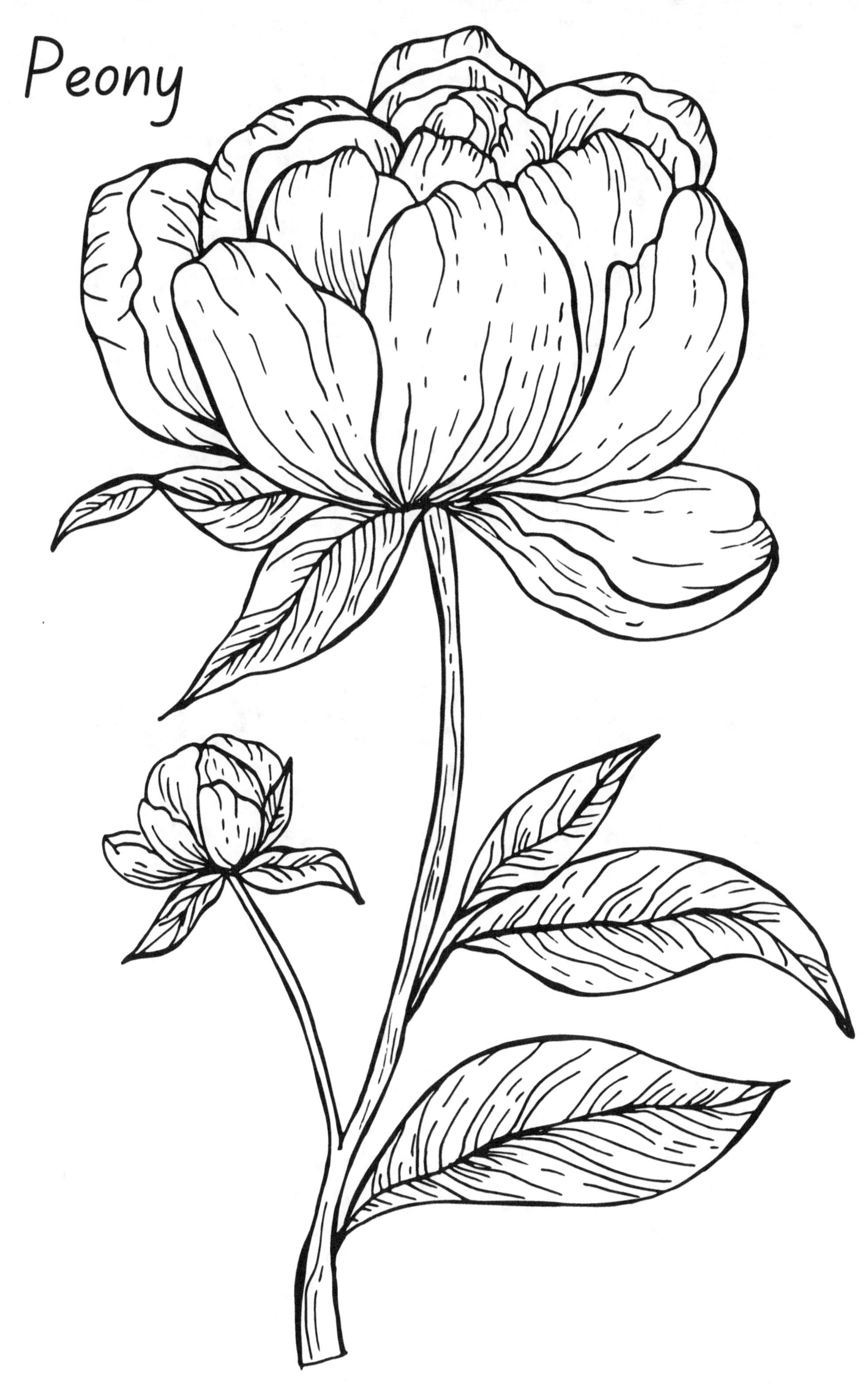

Take chances

Rose

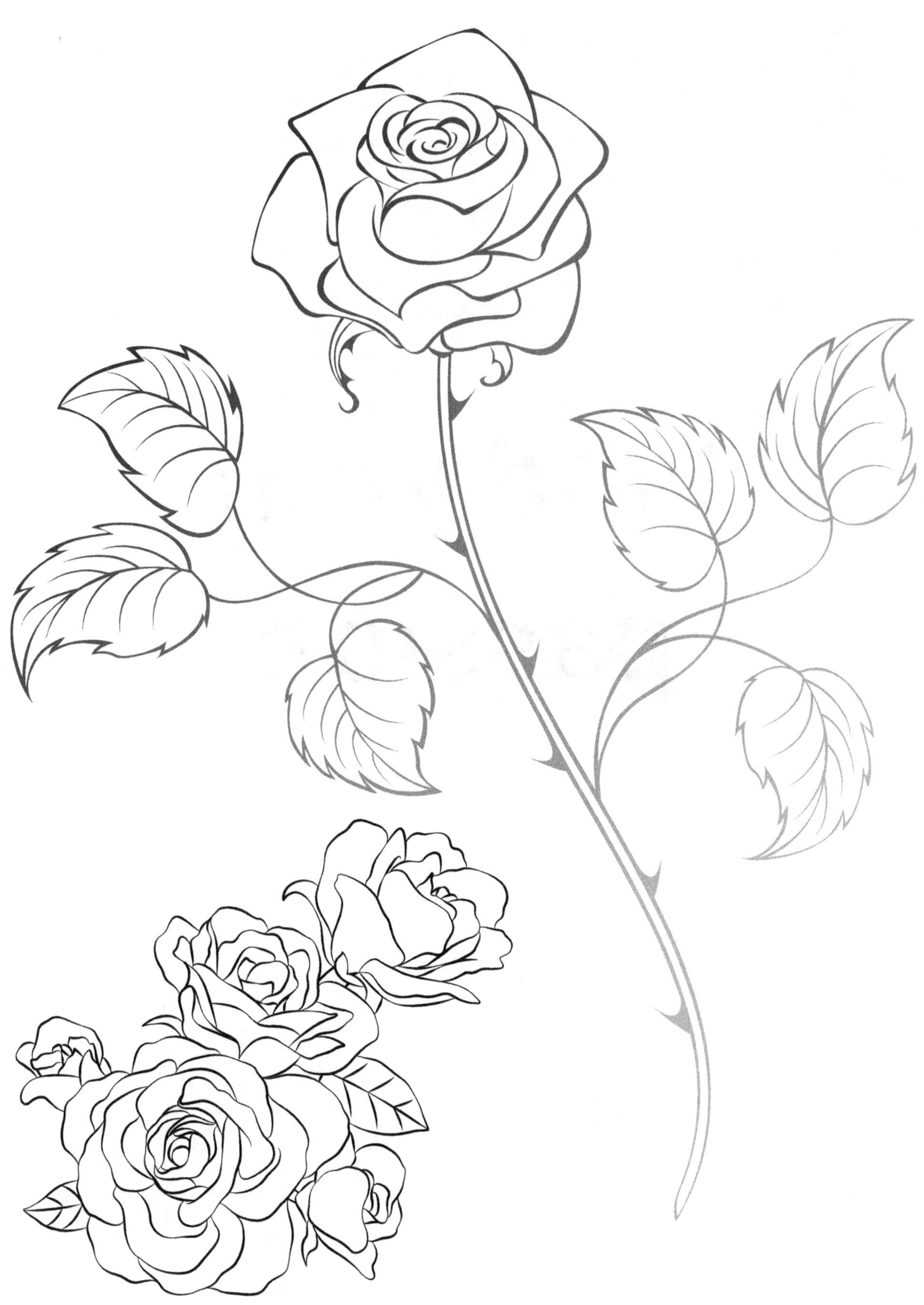

Find your passion

Tulips

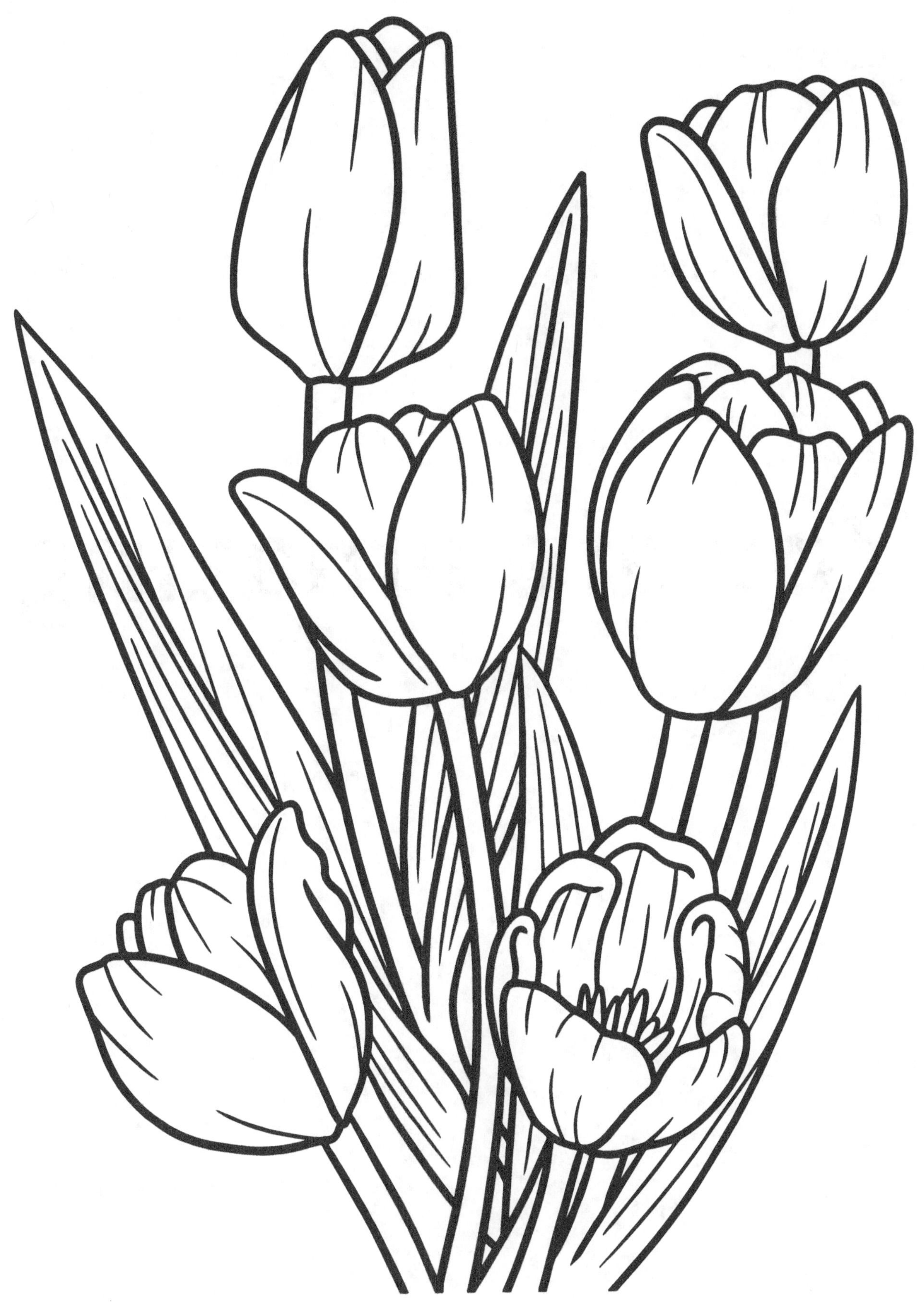

You are amazing

Flower Art

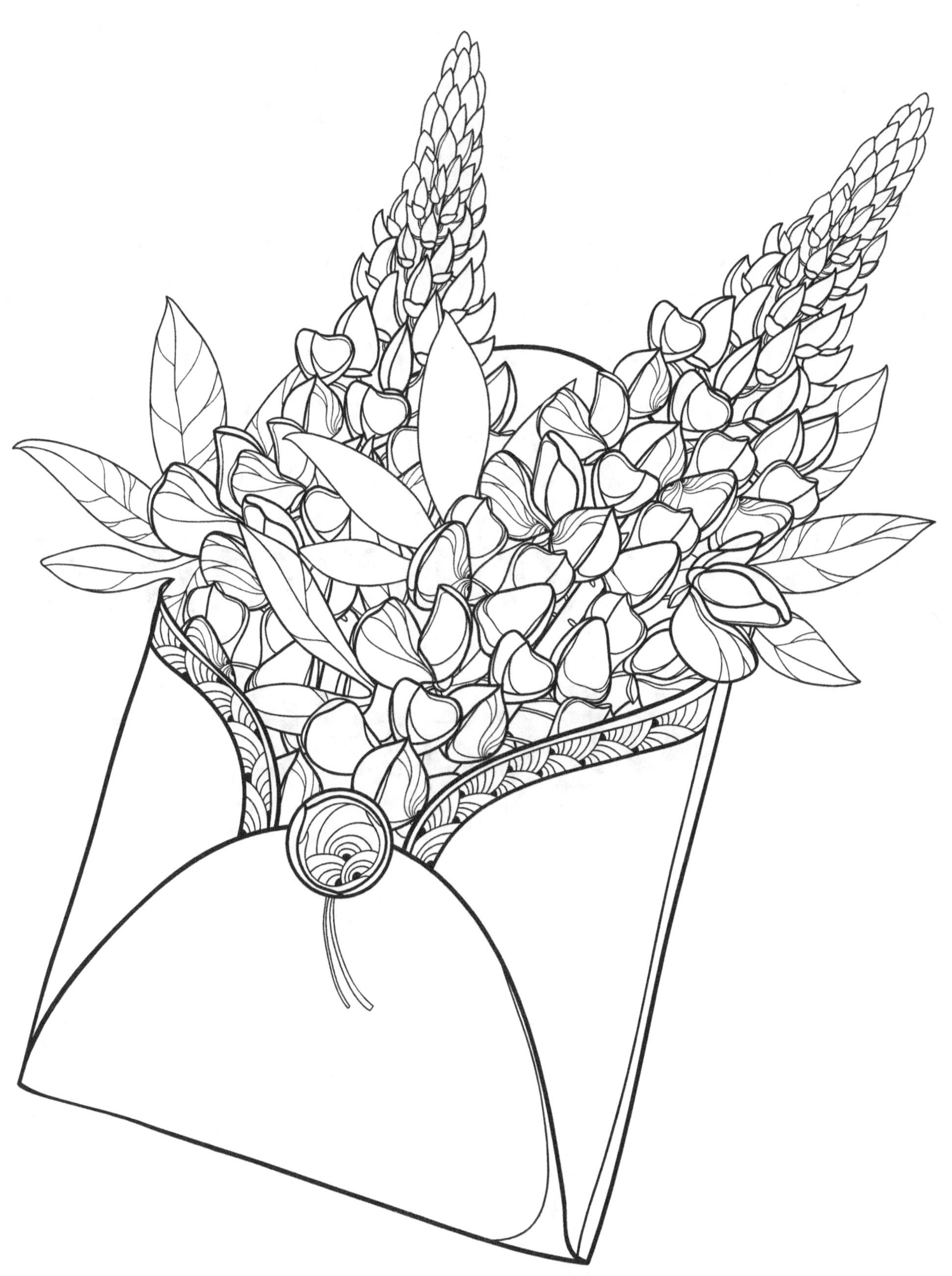

Clear your mind
of can't

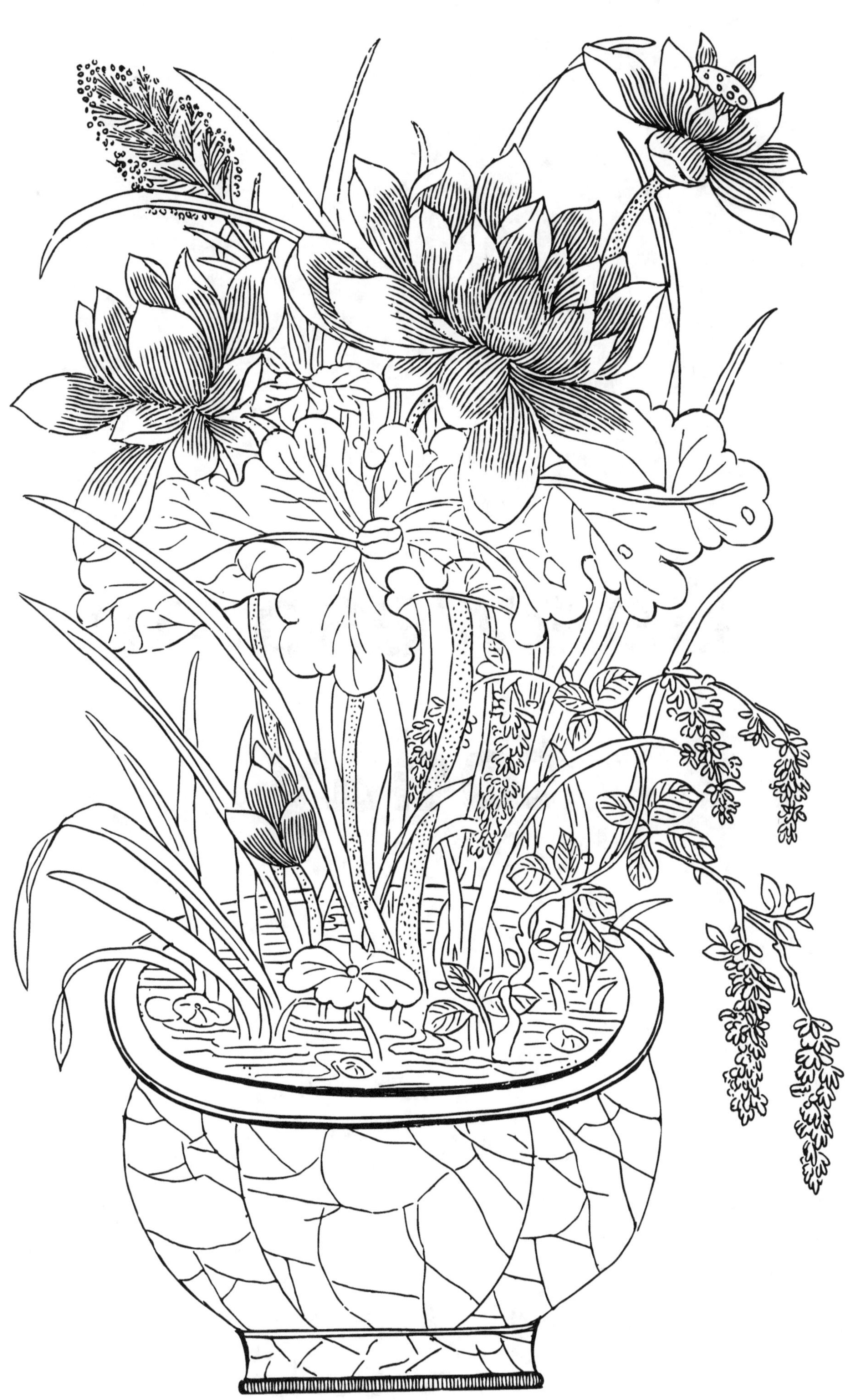

Be awesome today

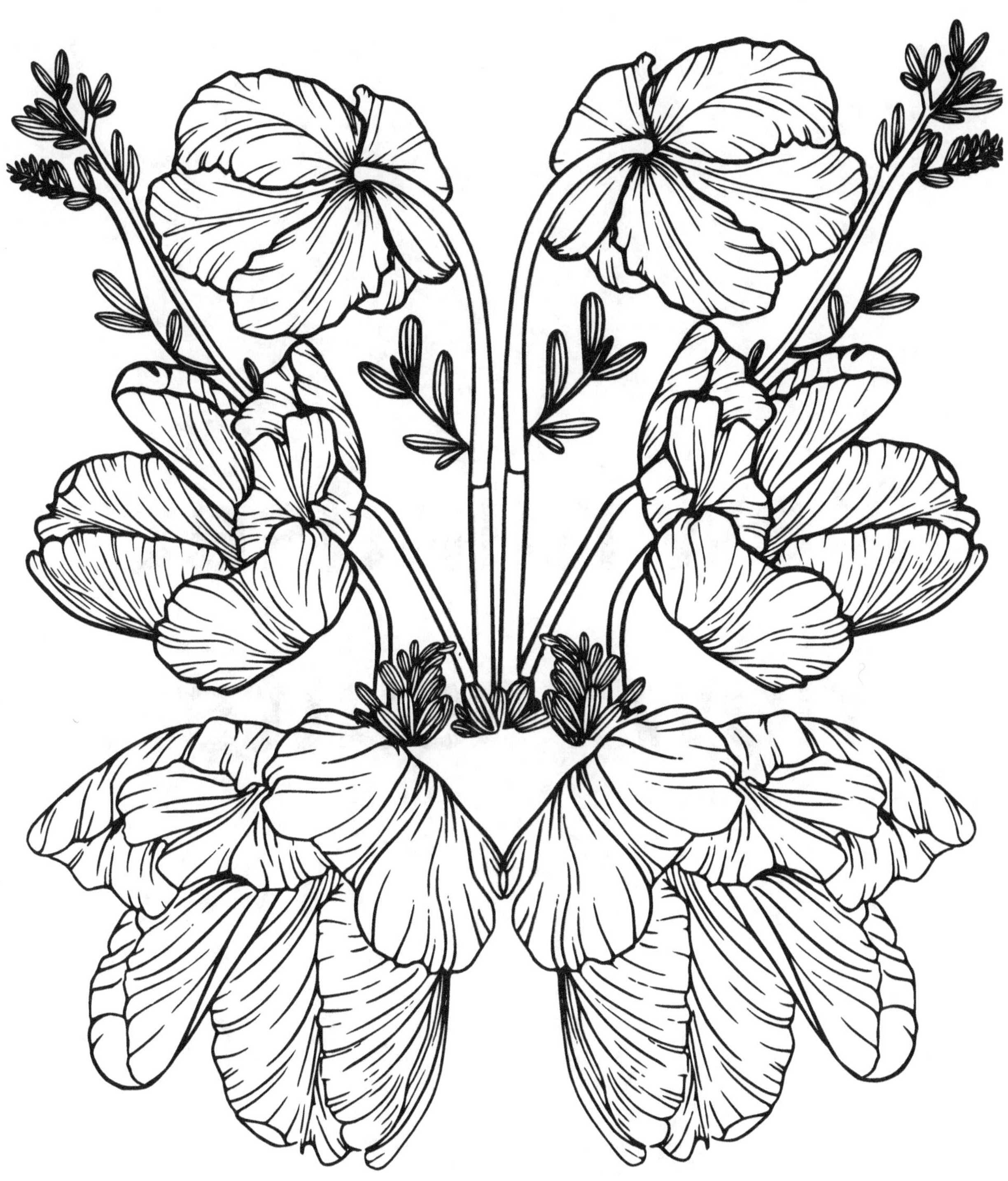

New mindset
new results

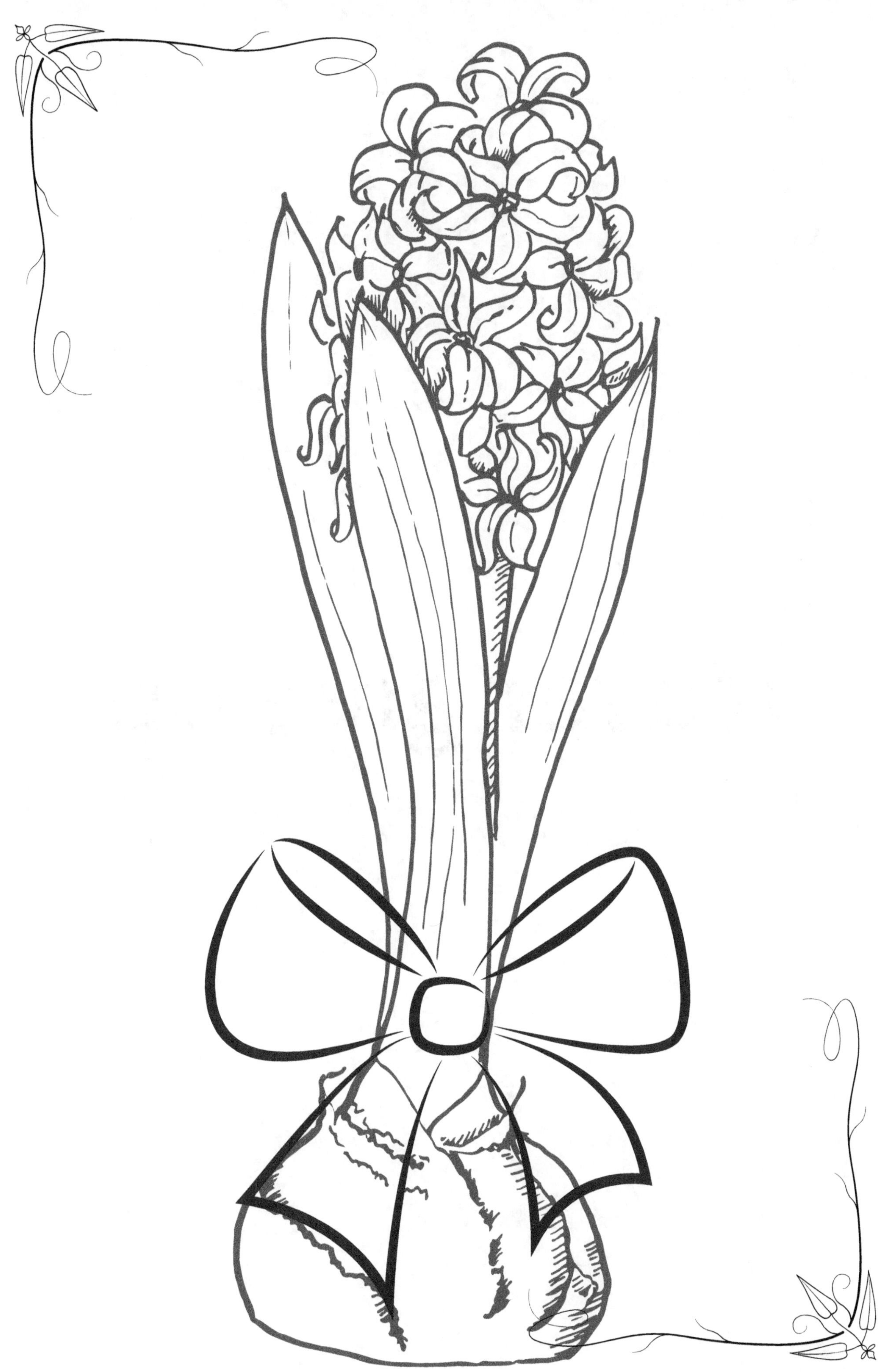

Never give up

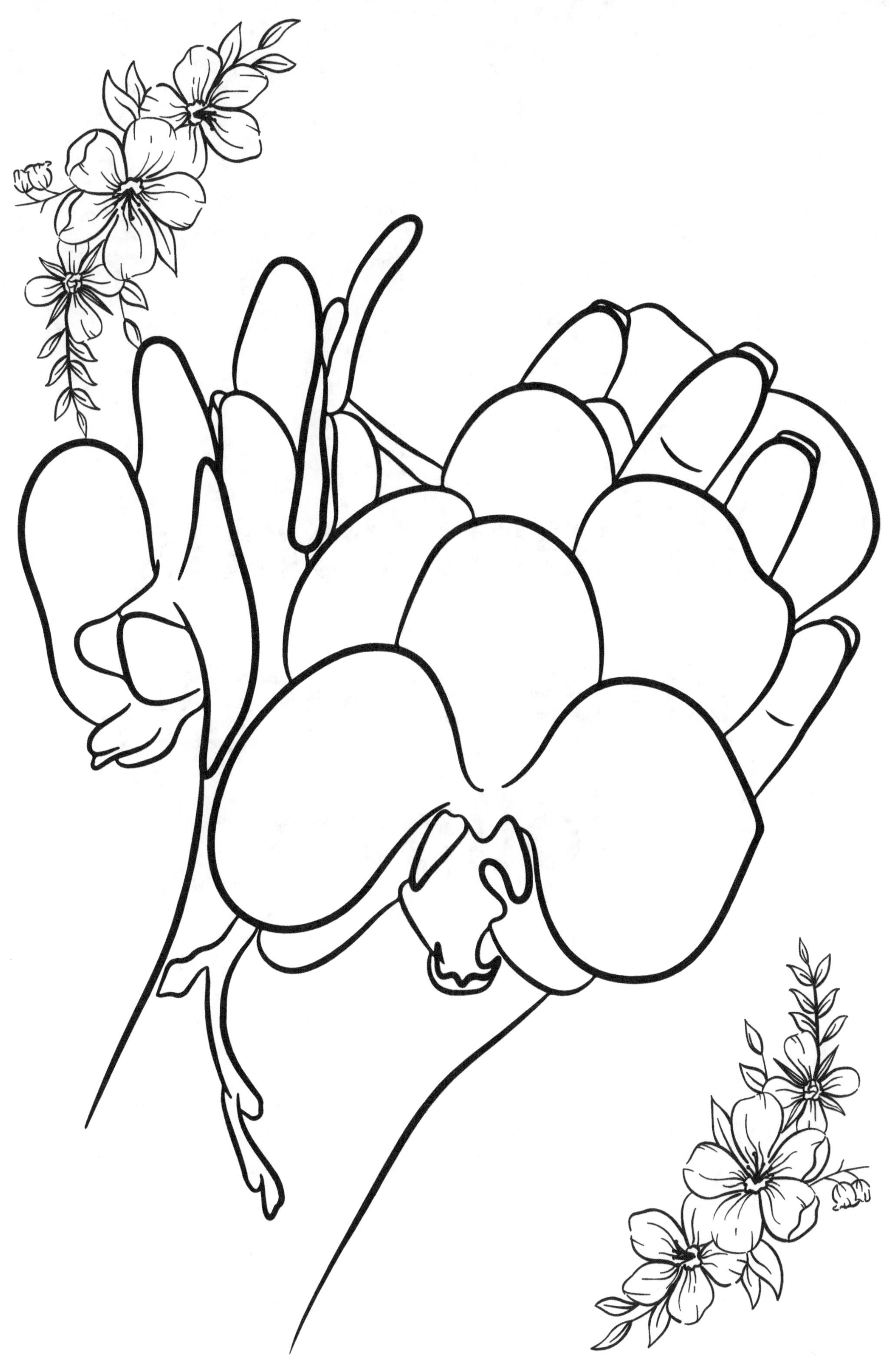

Where focus goes energy follows

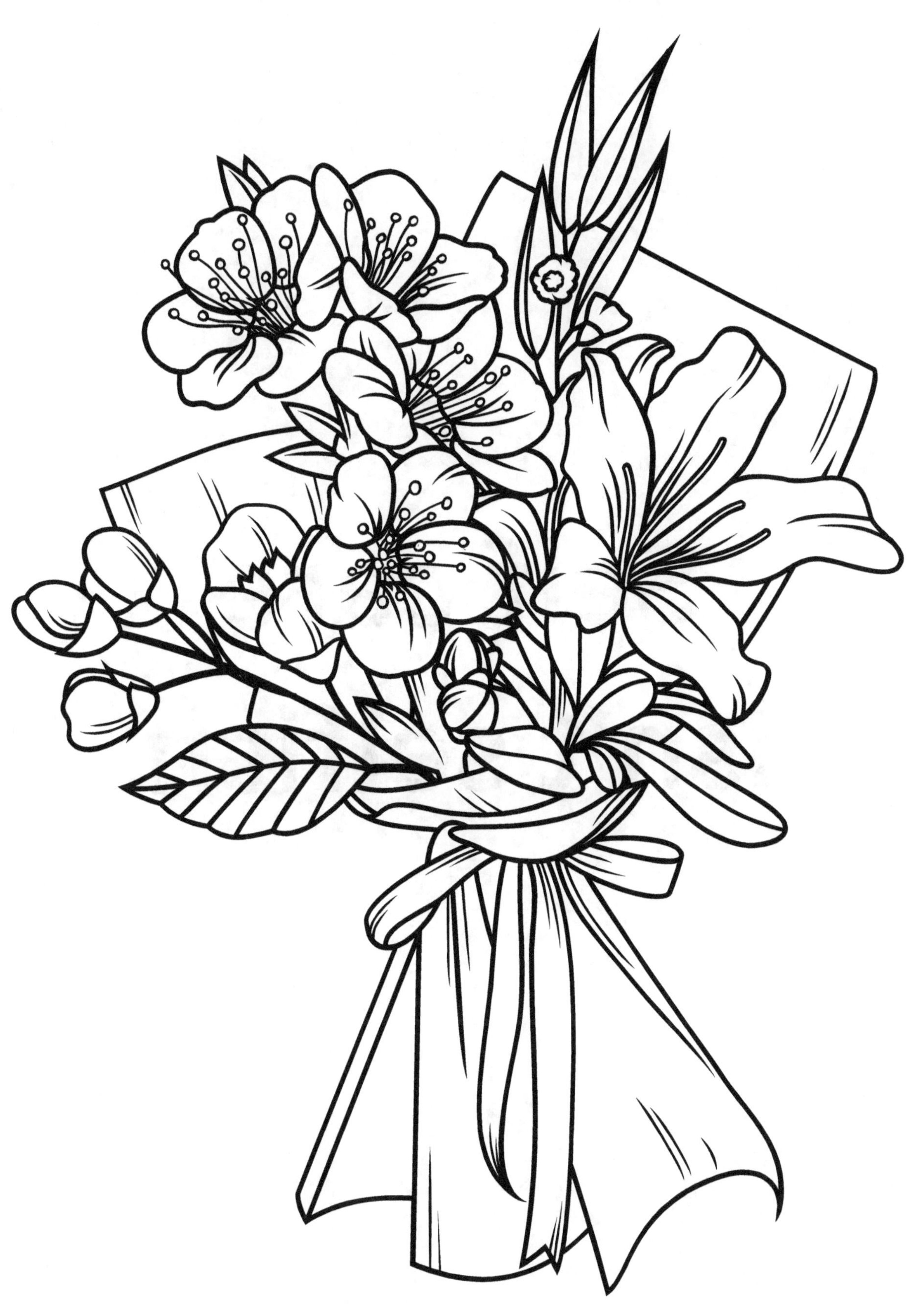

Self care
isn't selfish

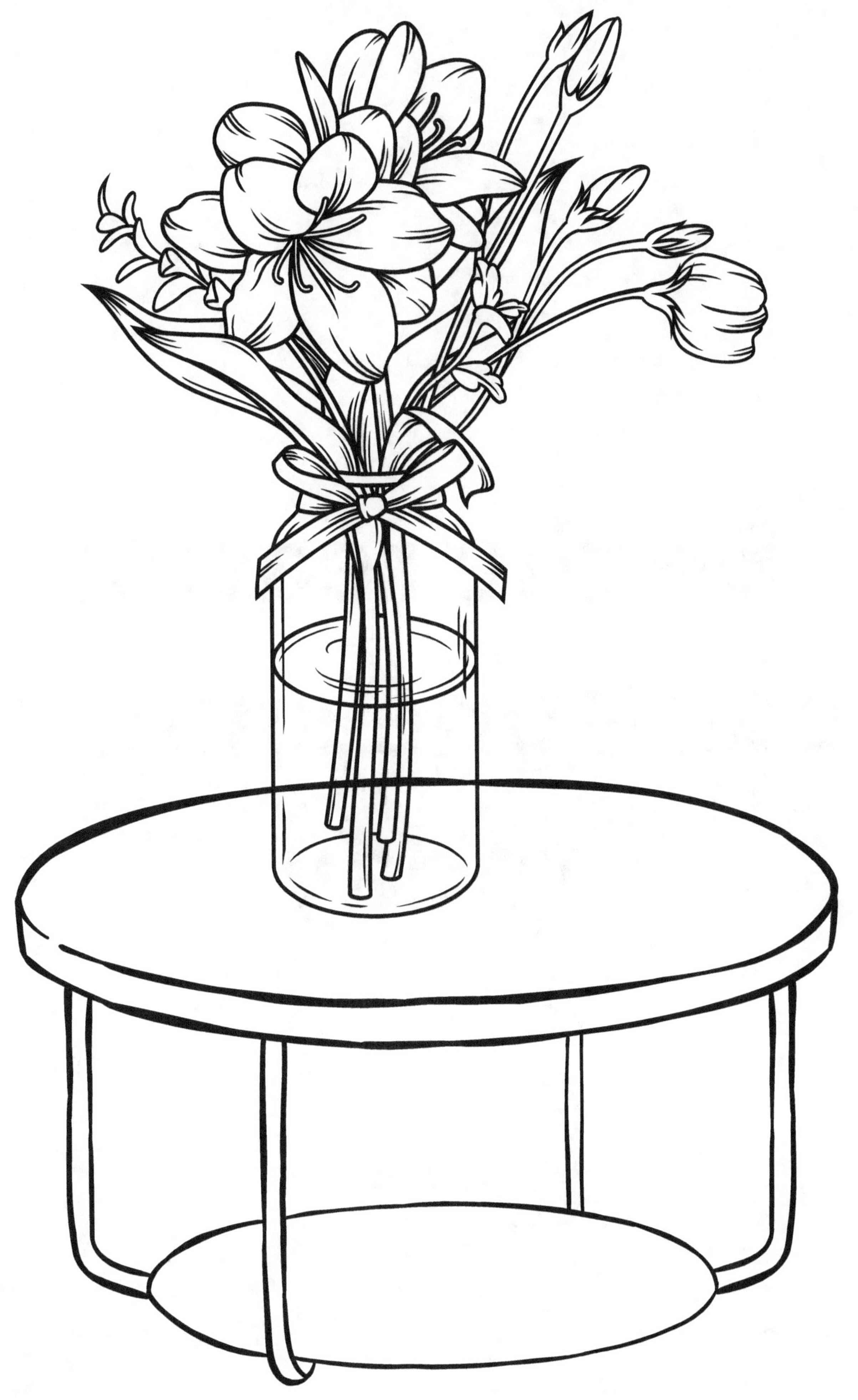

Be the reason someone smiles today

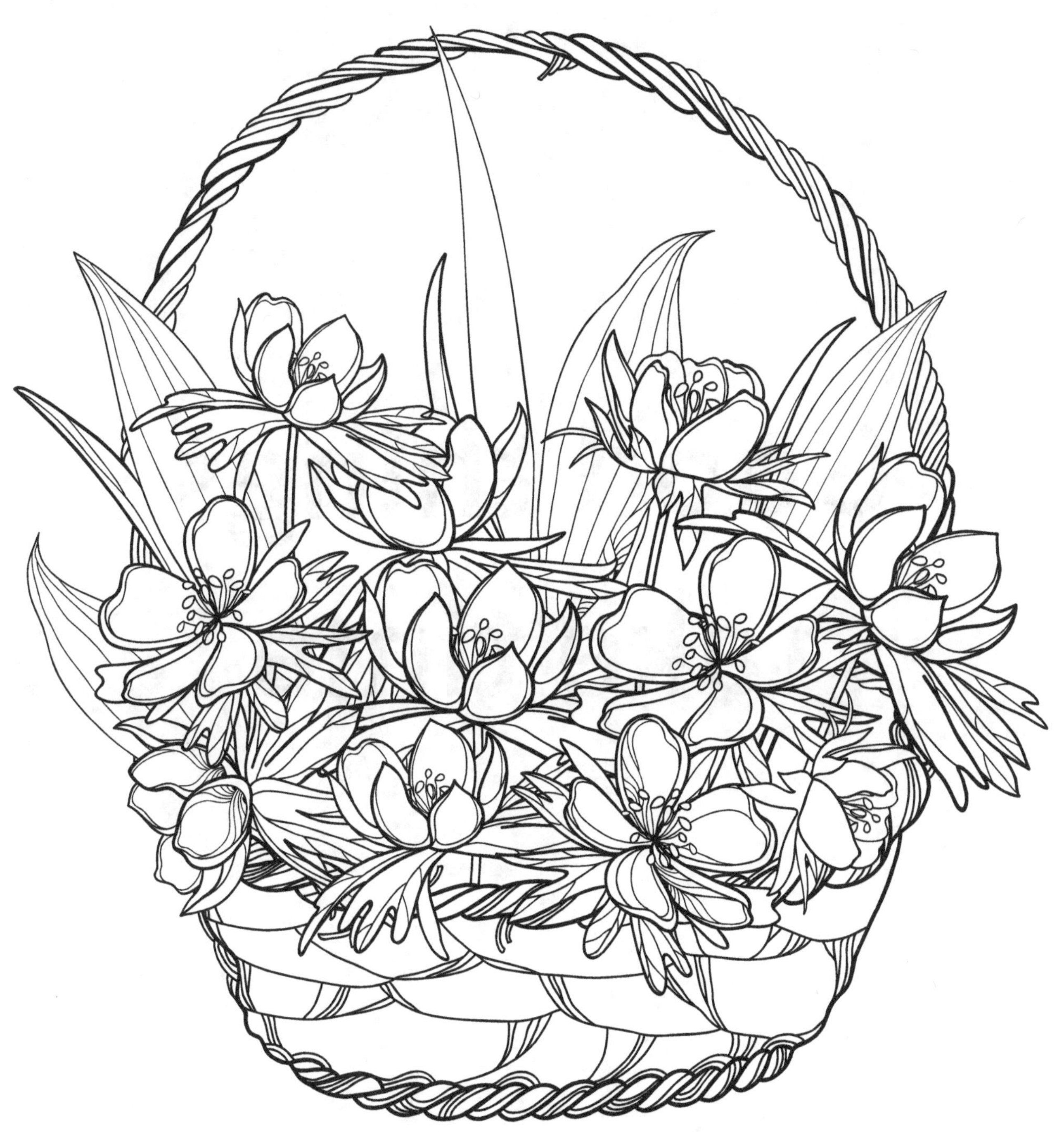

Good things take time

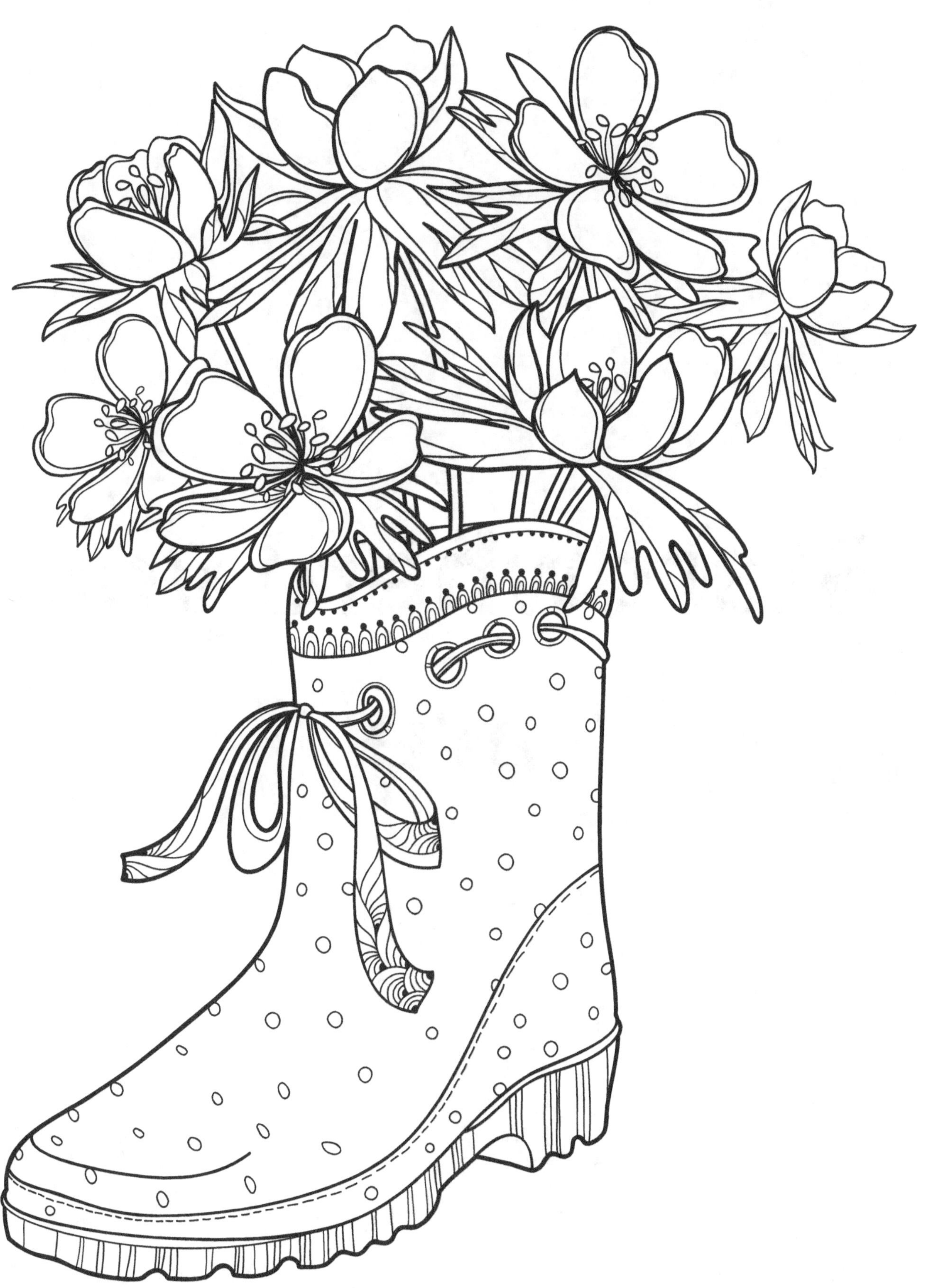

Start where you are

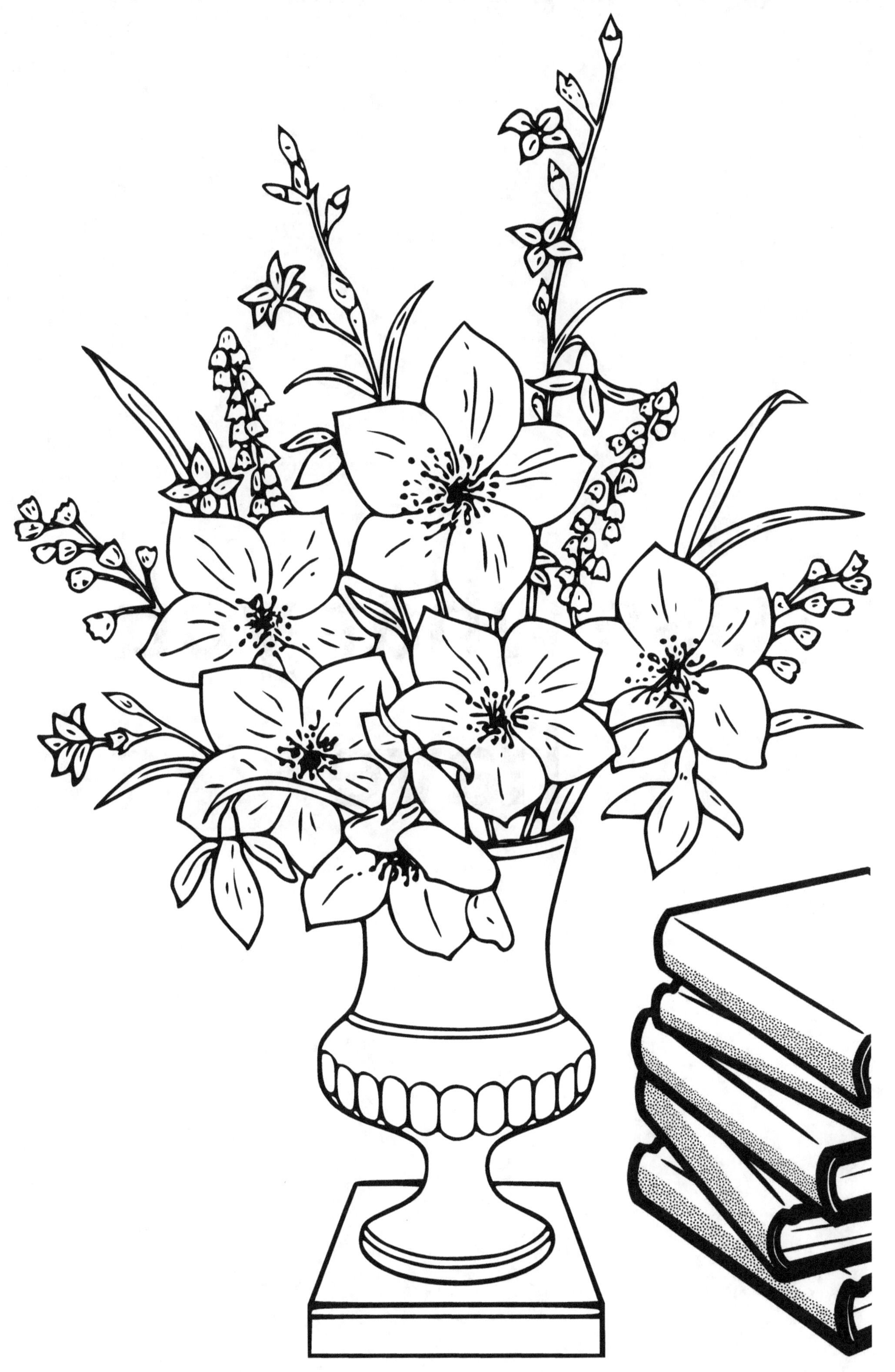

Use what you have

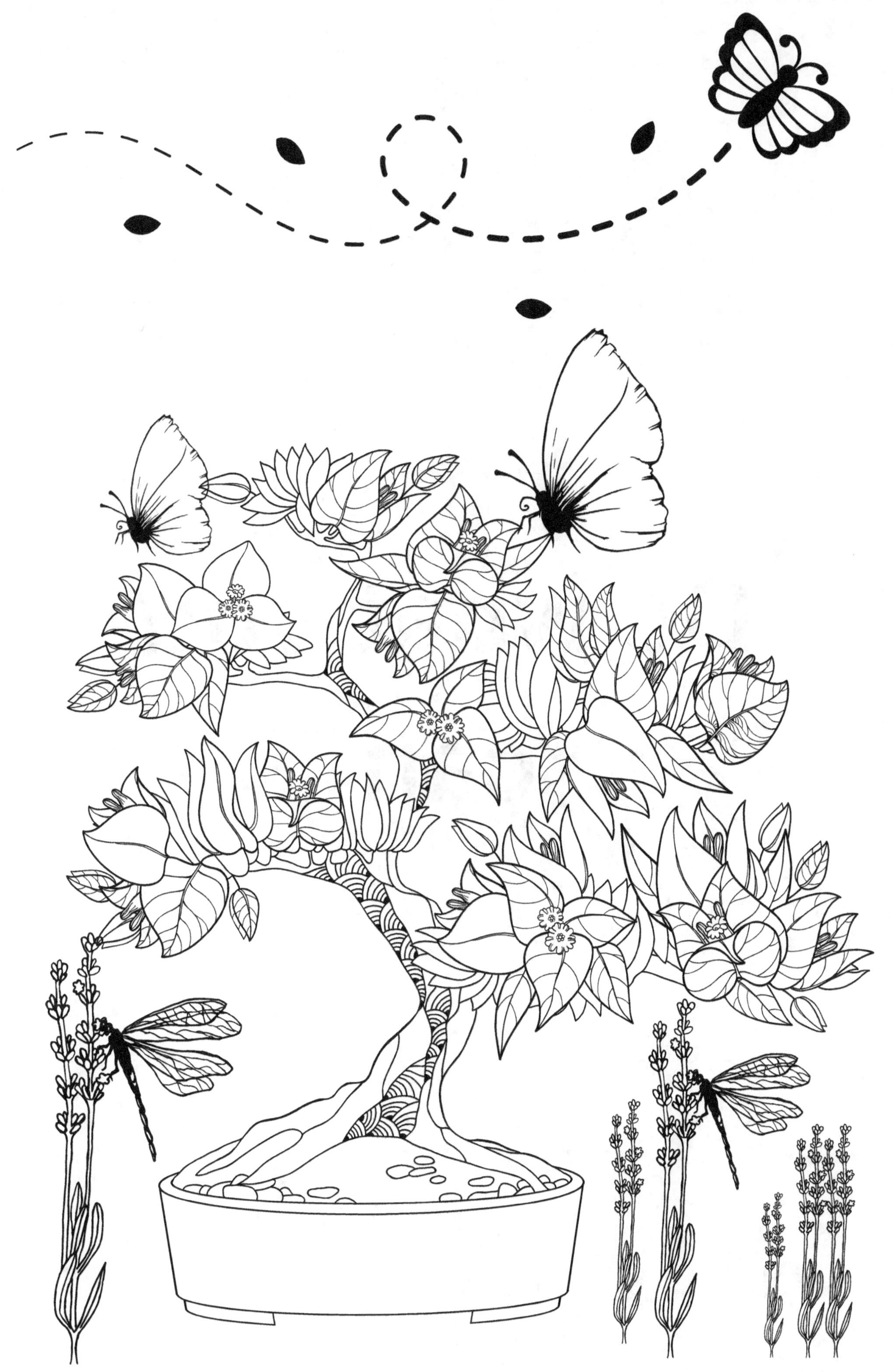

Do what you
can

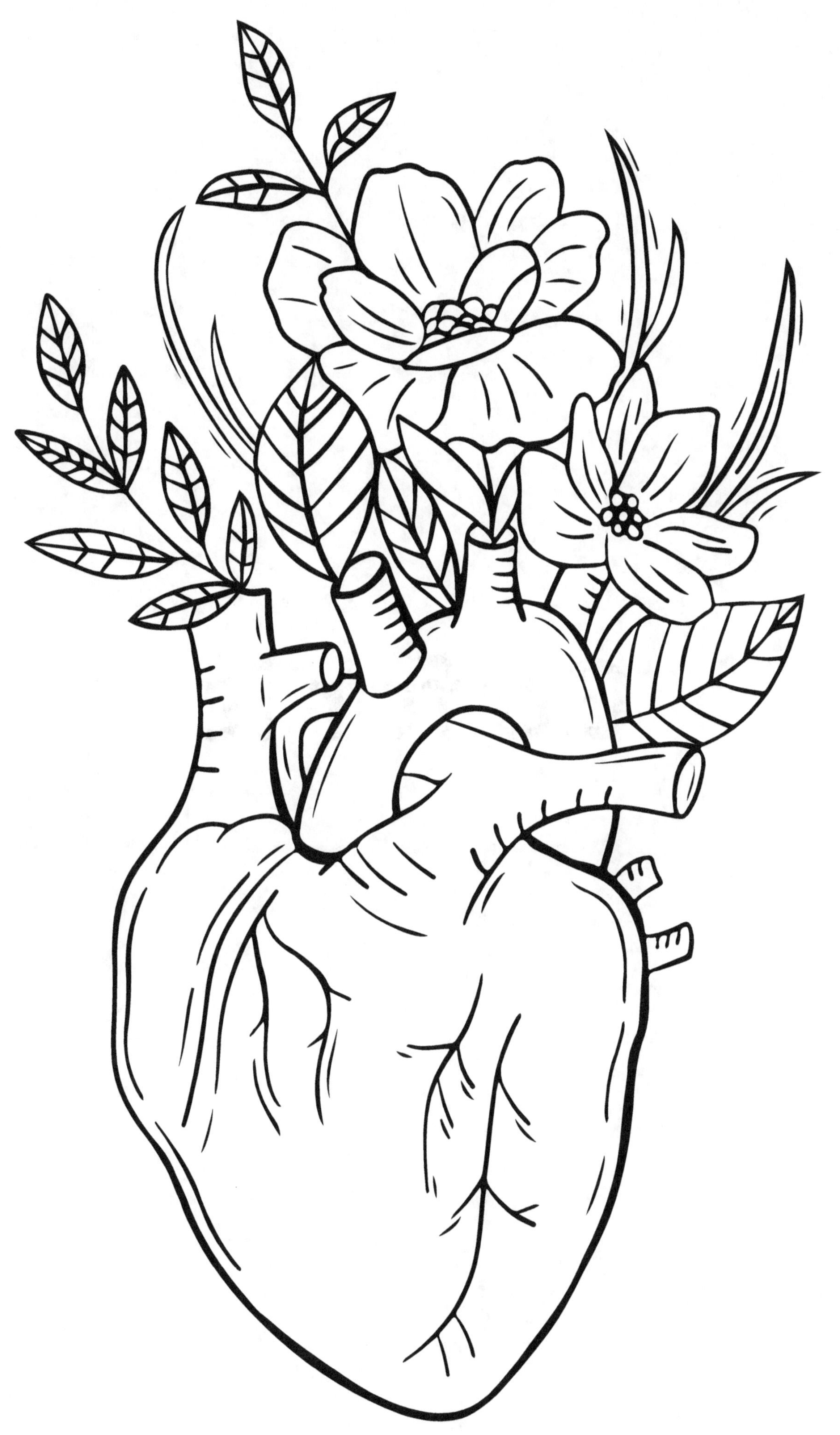

Go for it

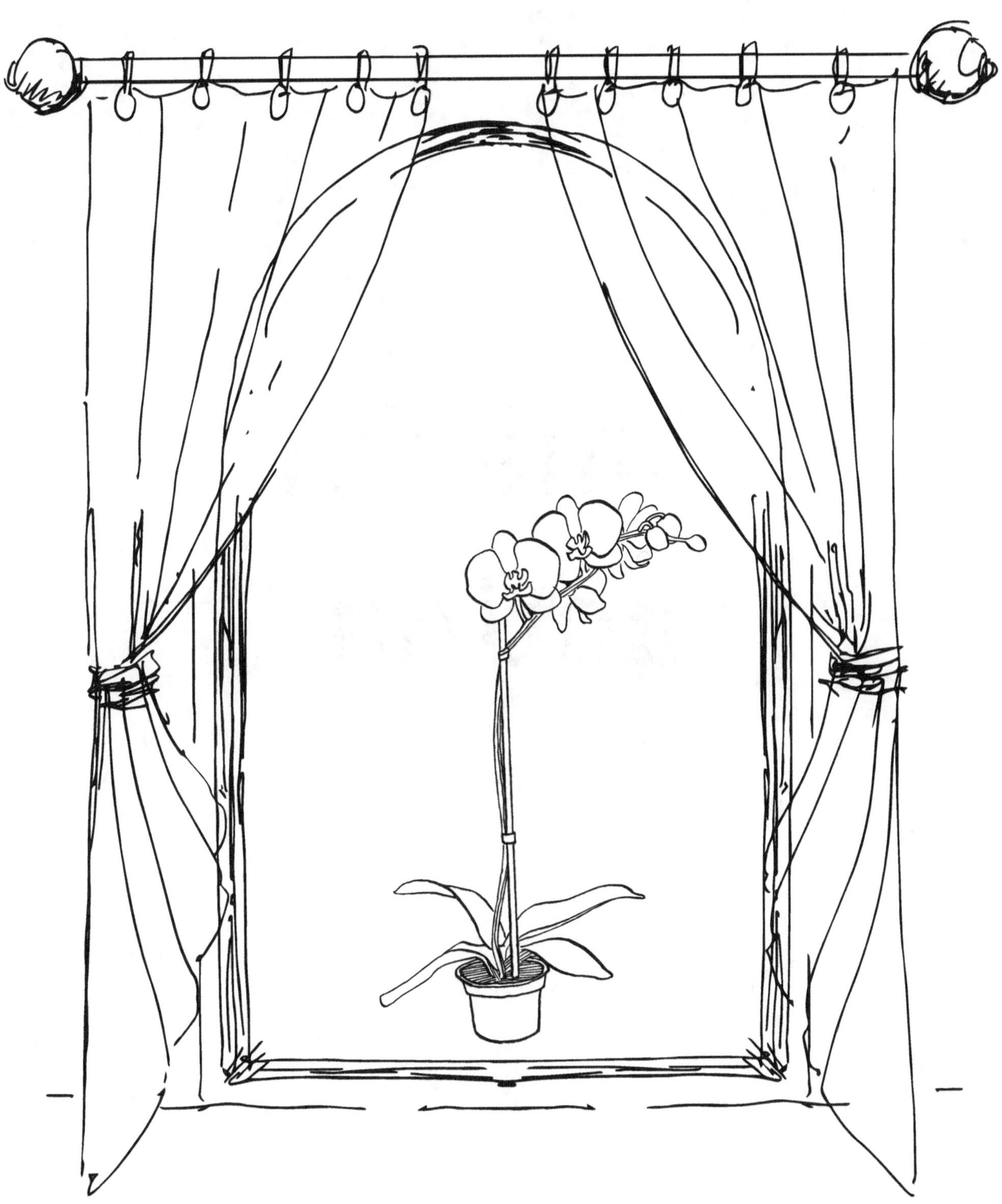

Time for
action

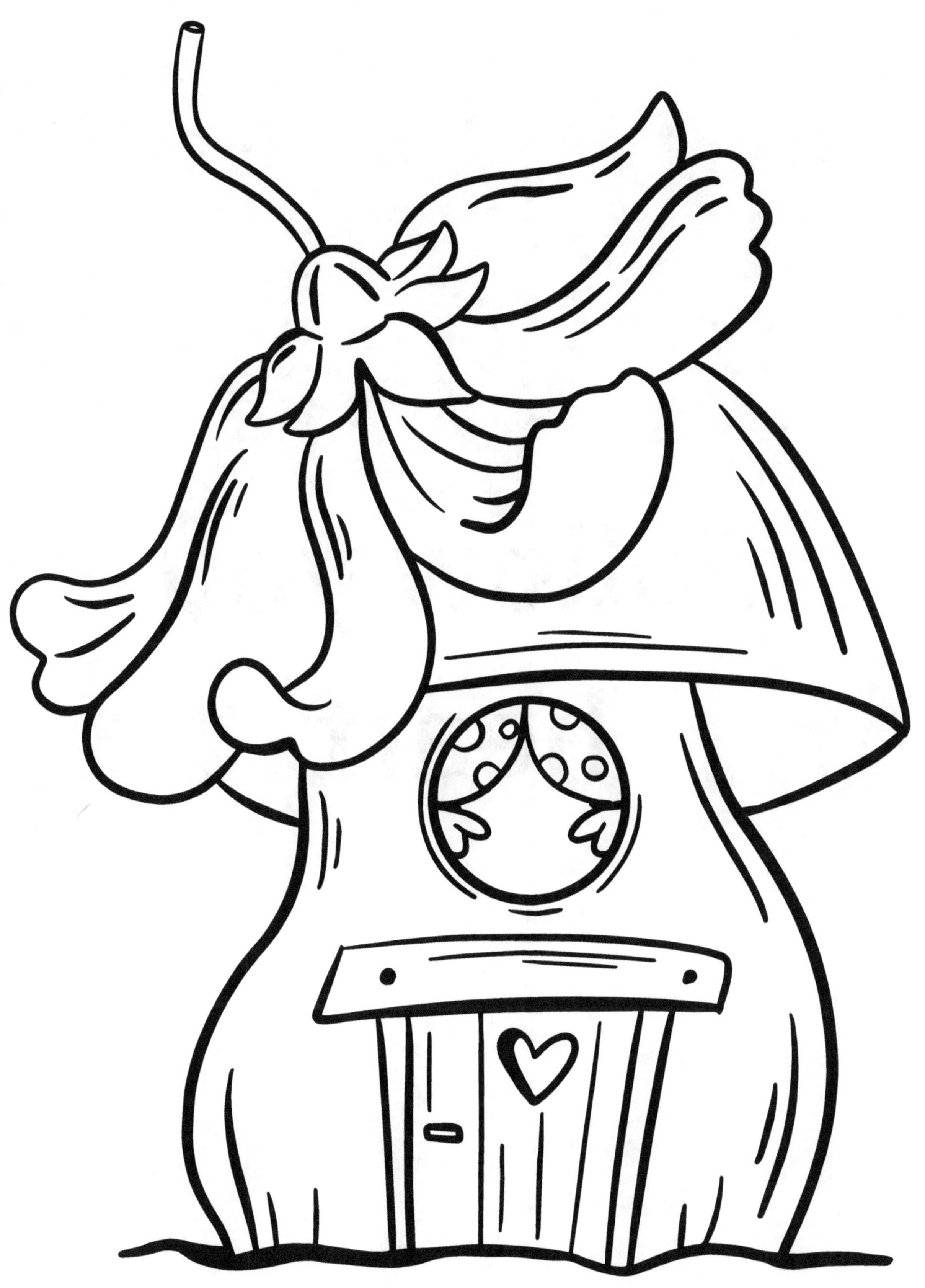

Follow you
heart

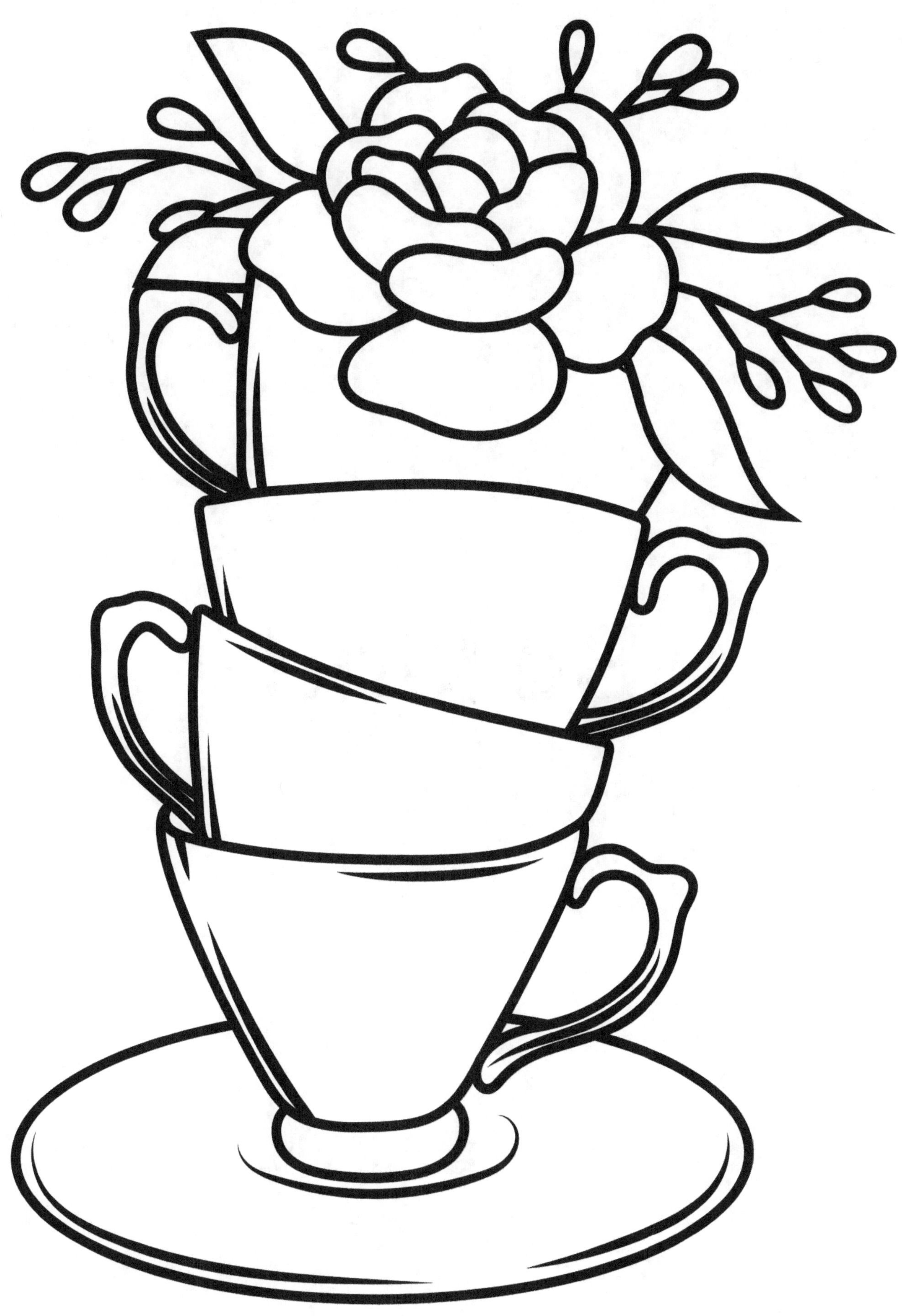

Be kind

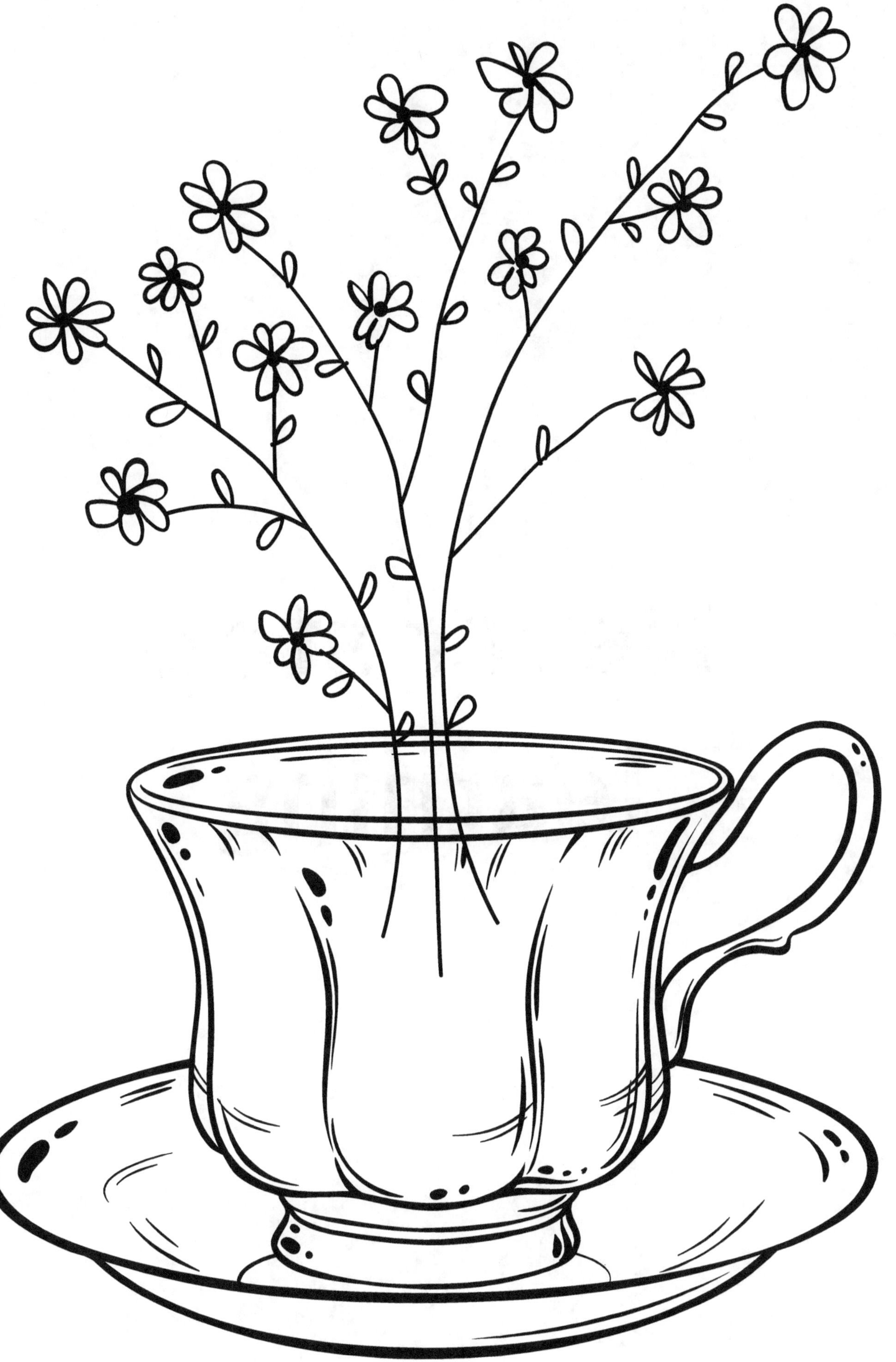

Never stop learning

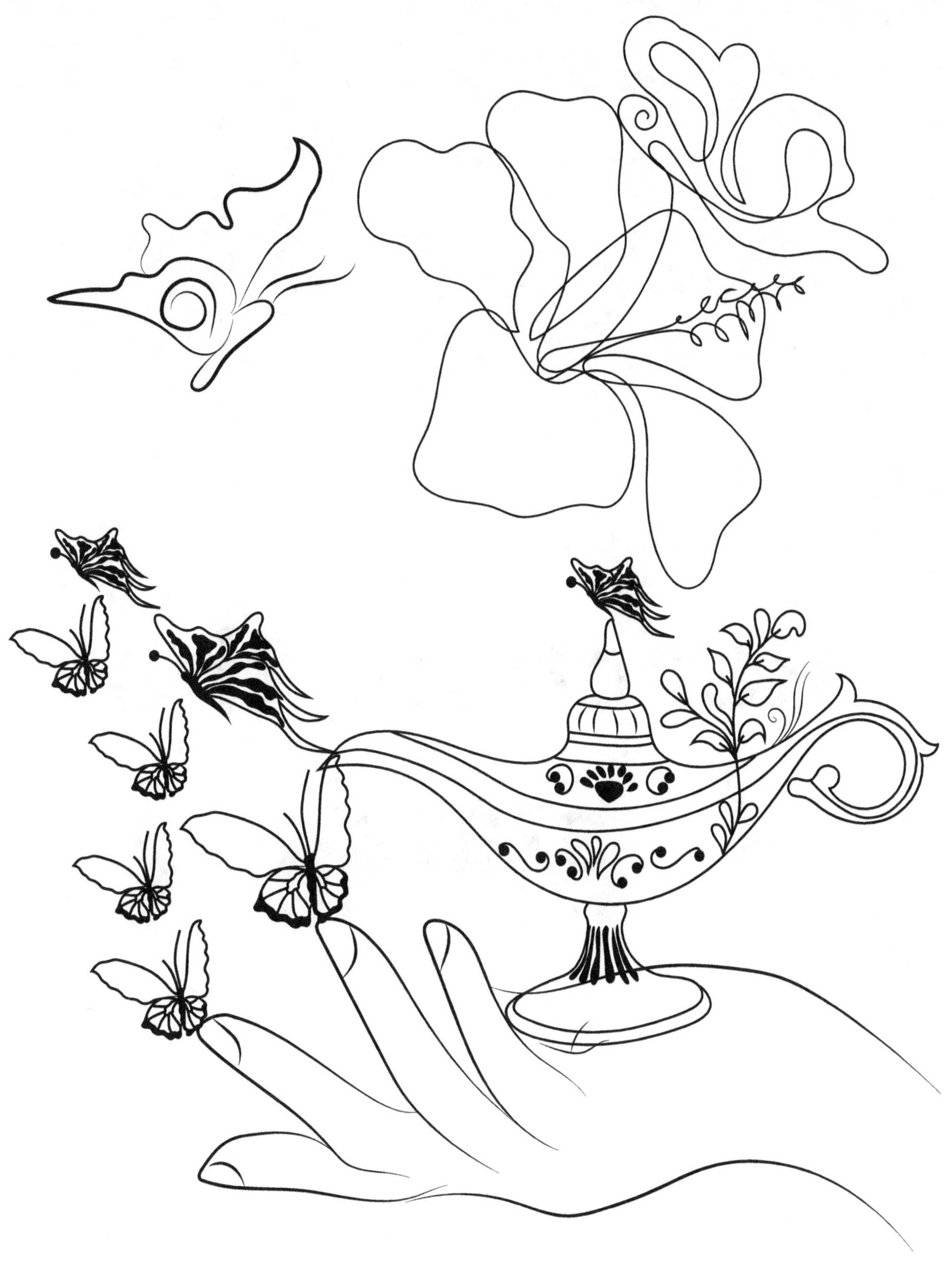

Reach for the stars

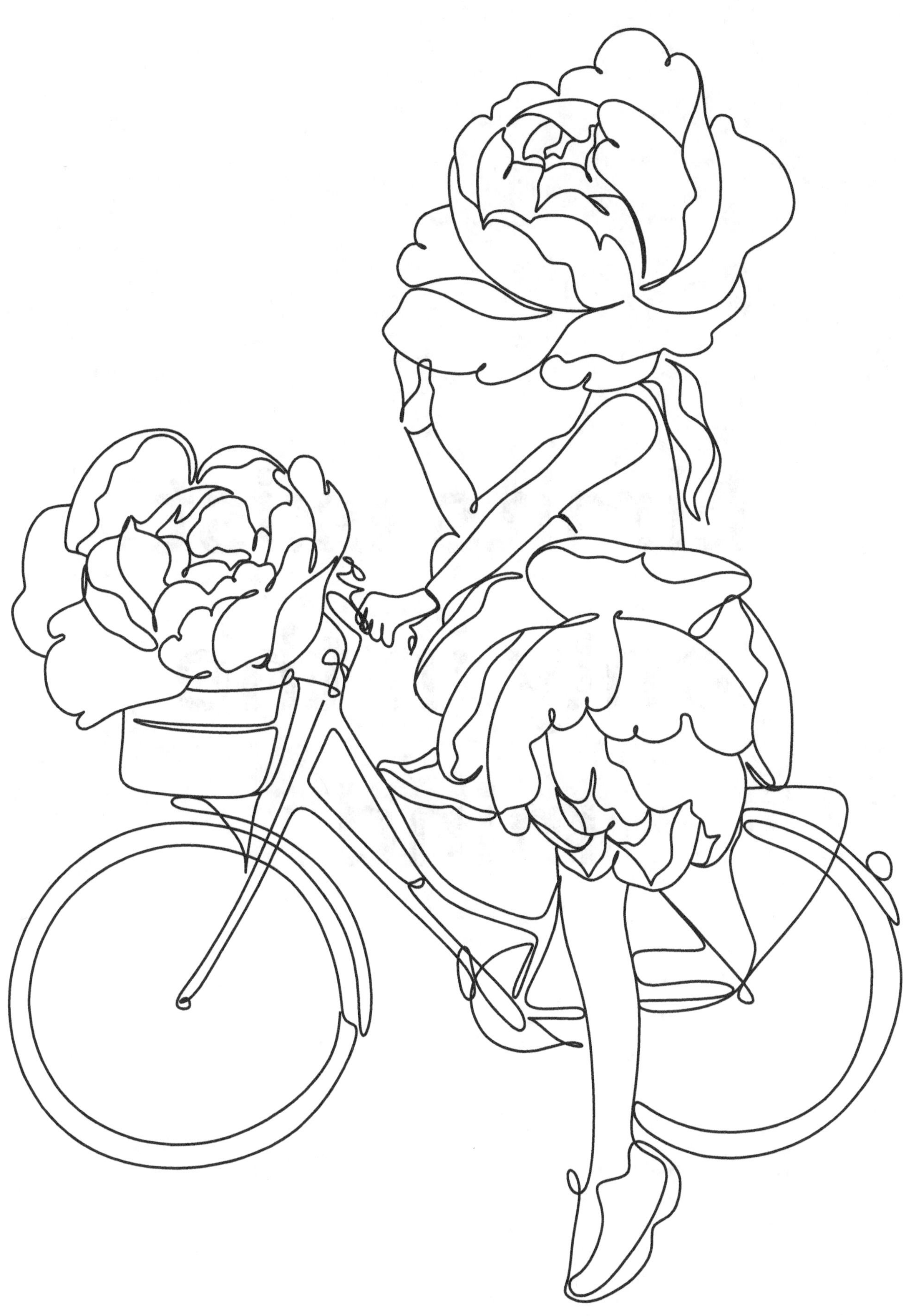

Limits exist only in the mind

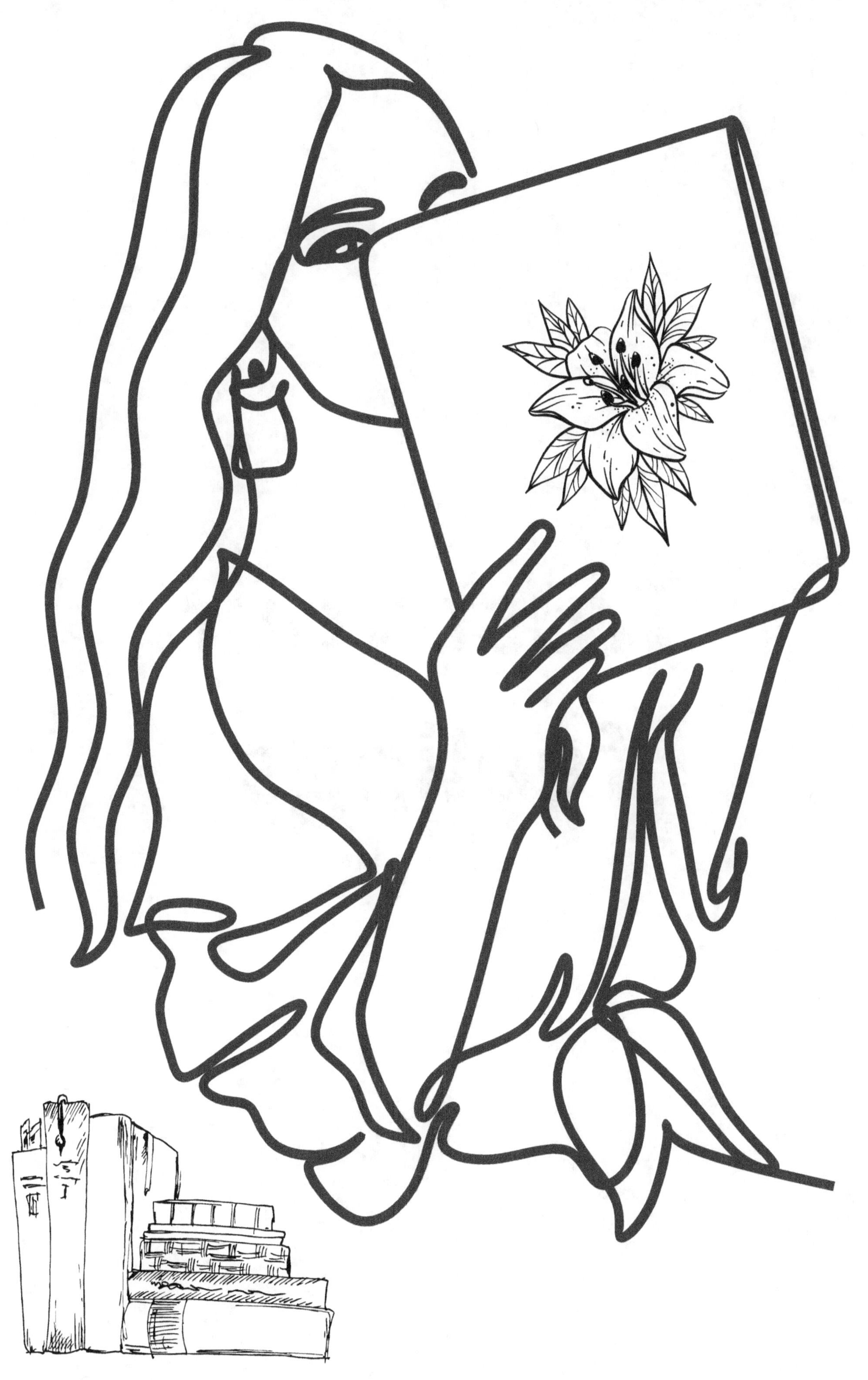

Trust your feelings

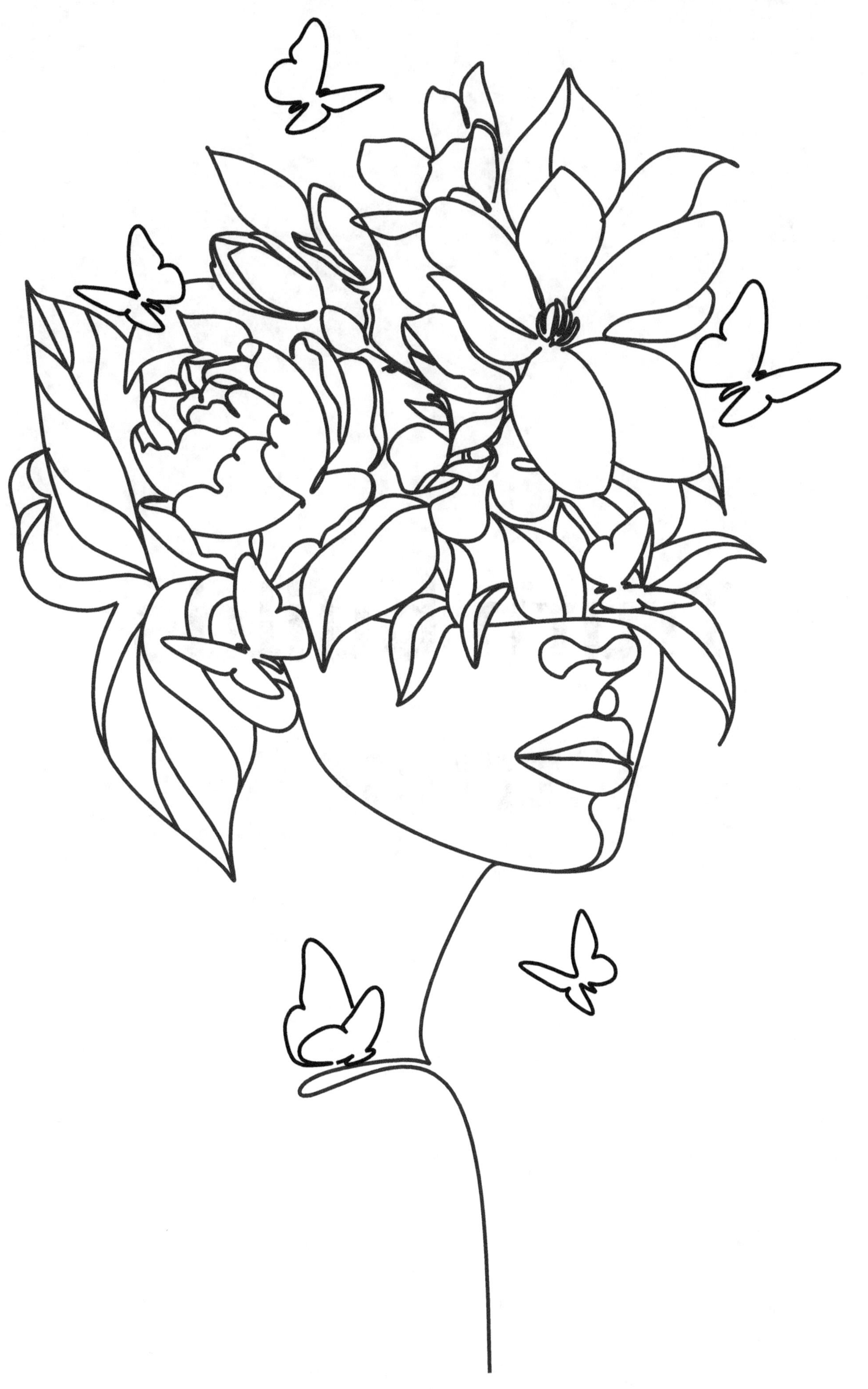

Truth builds trust

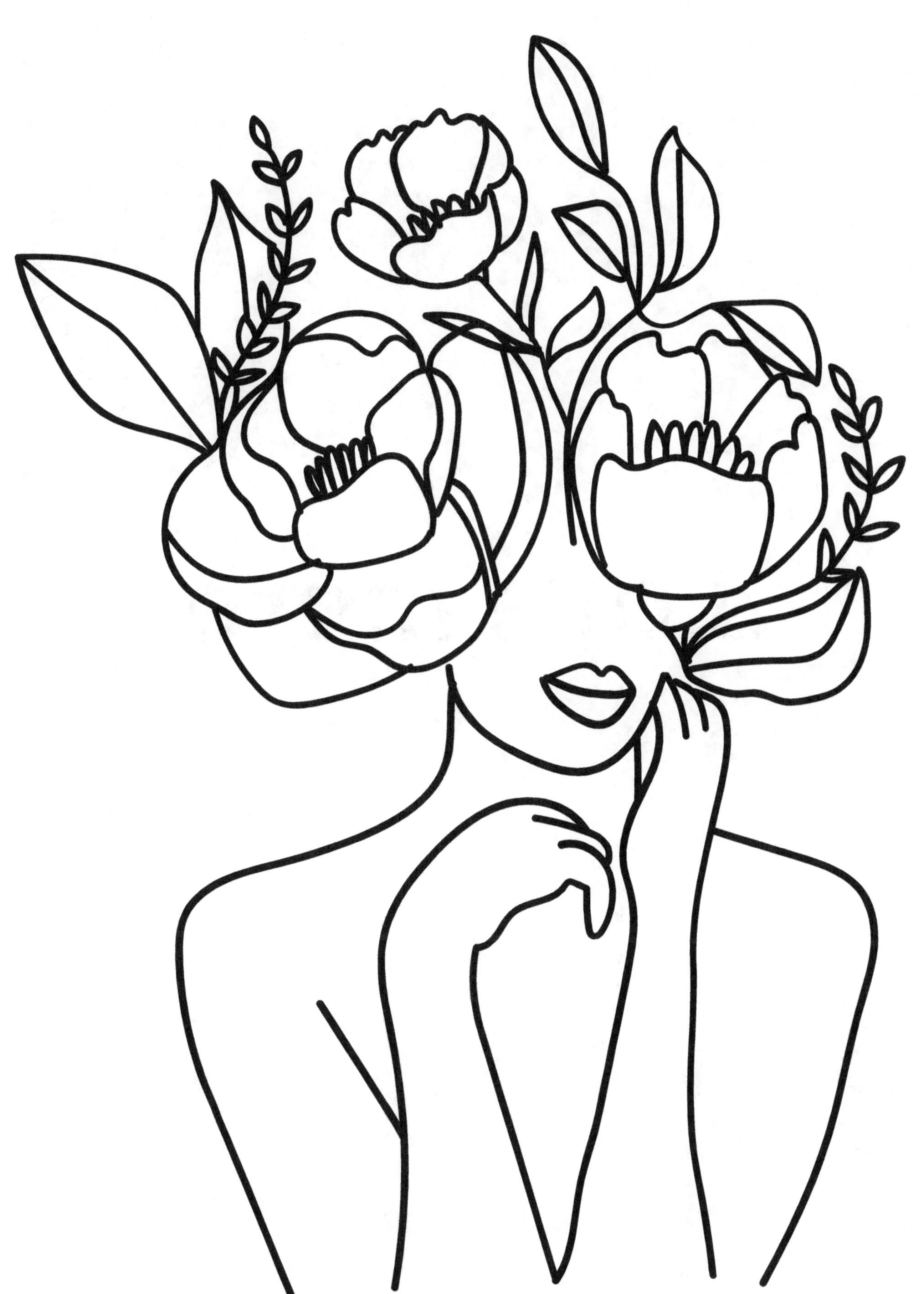

Love more

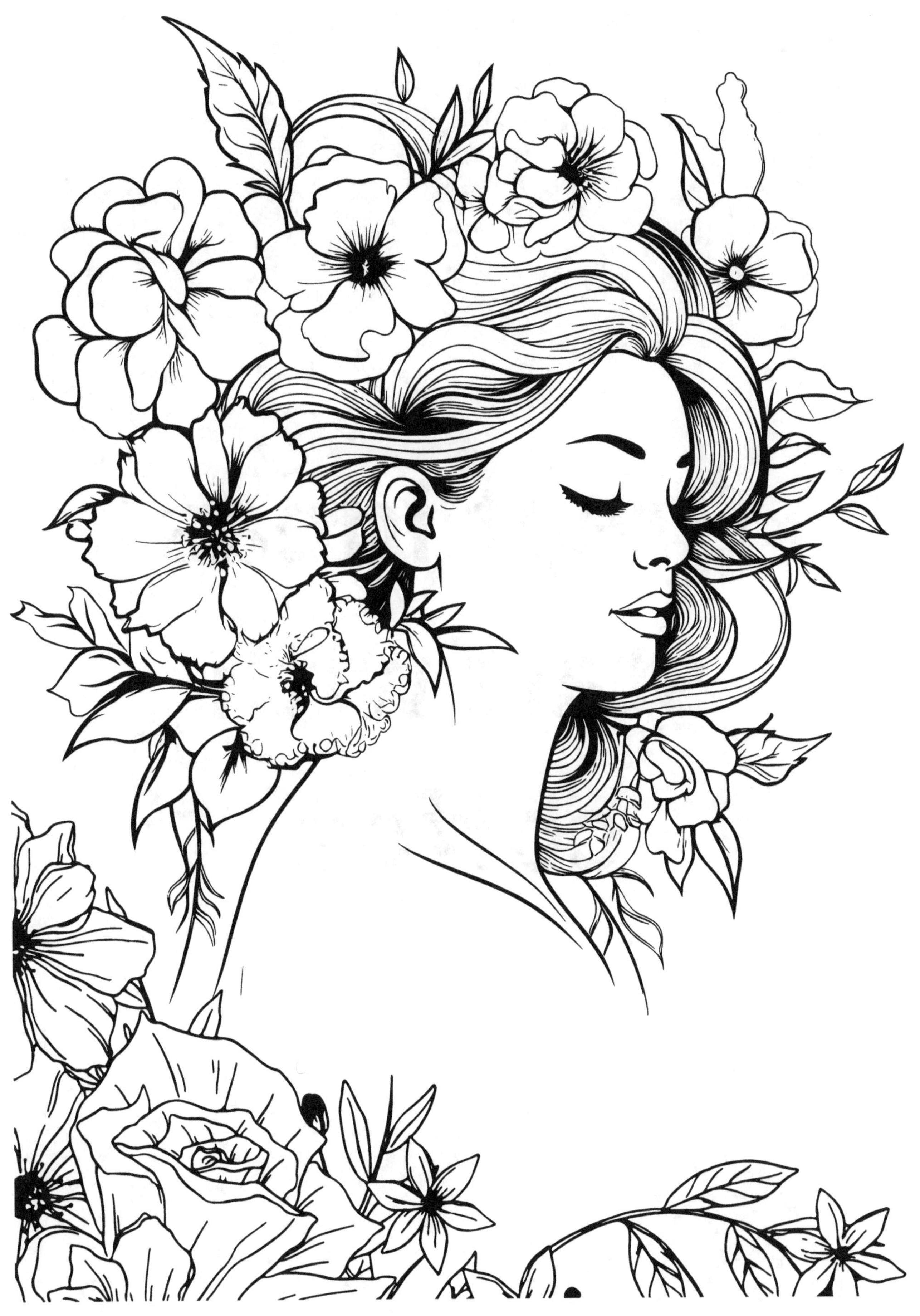

Great ideas start with coffee

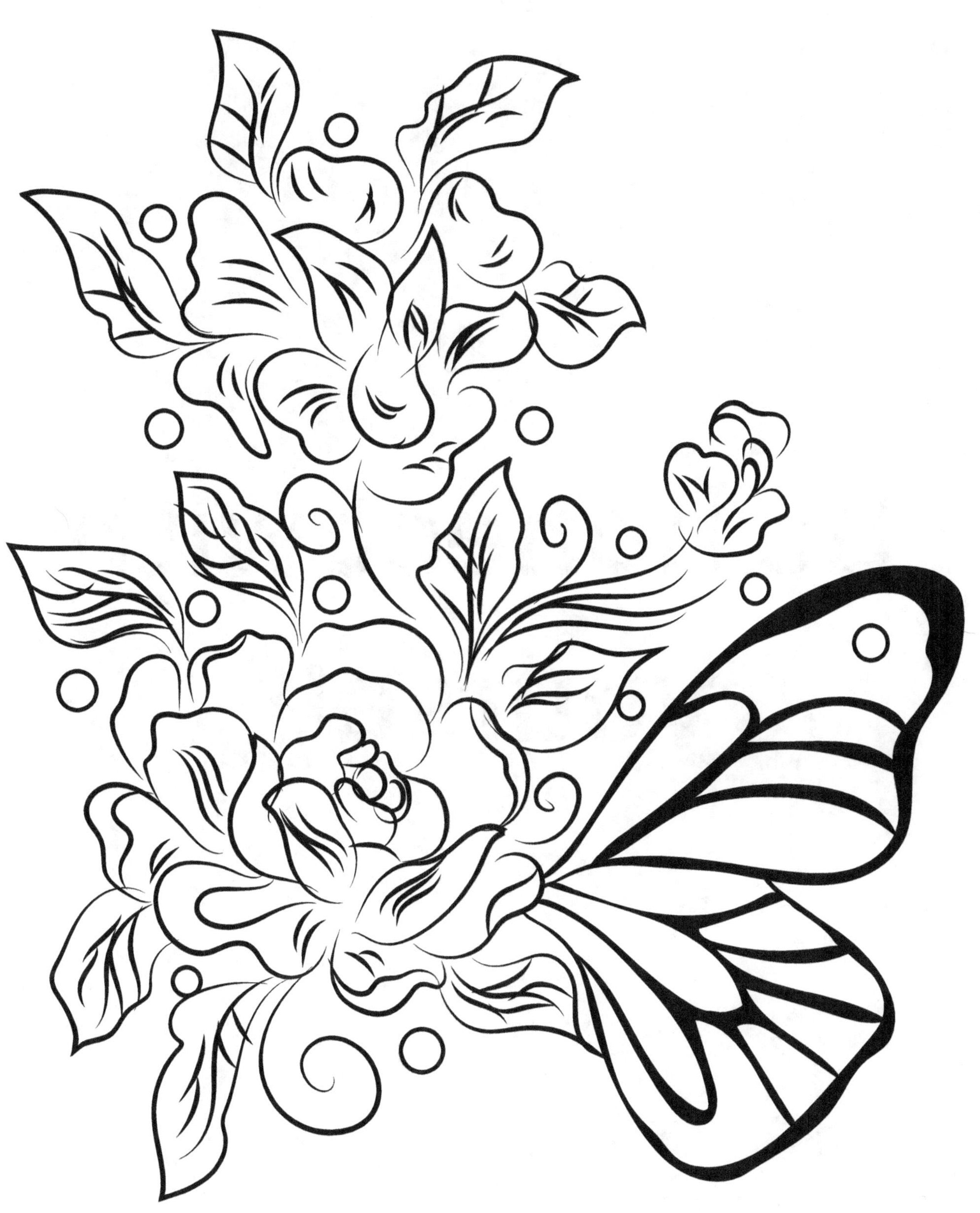

Be honest with yourself

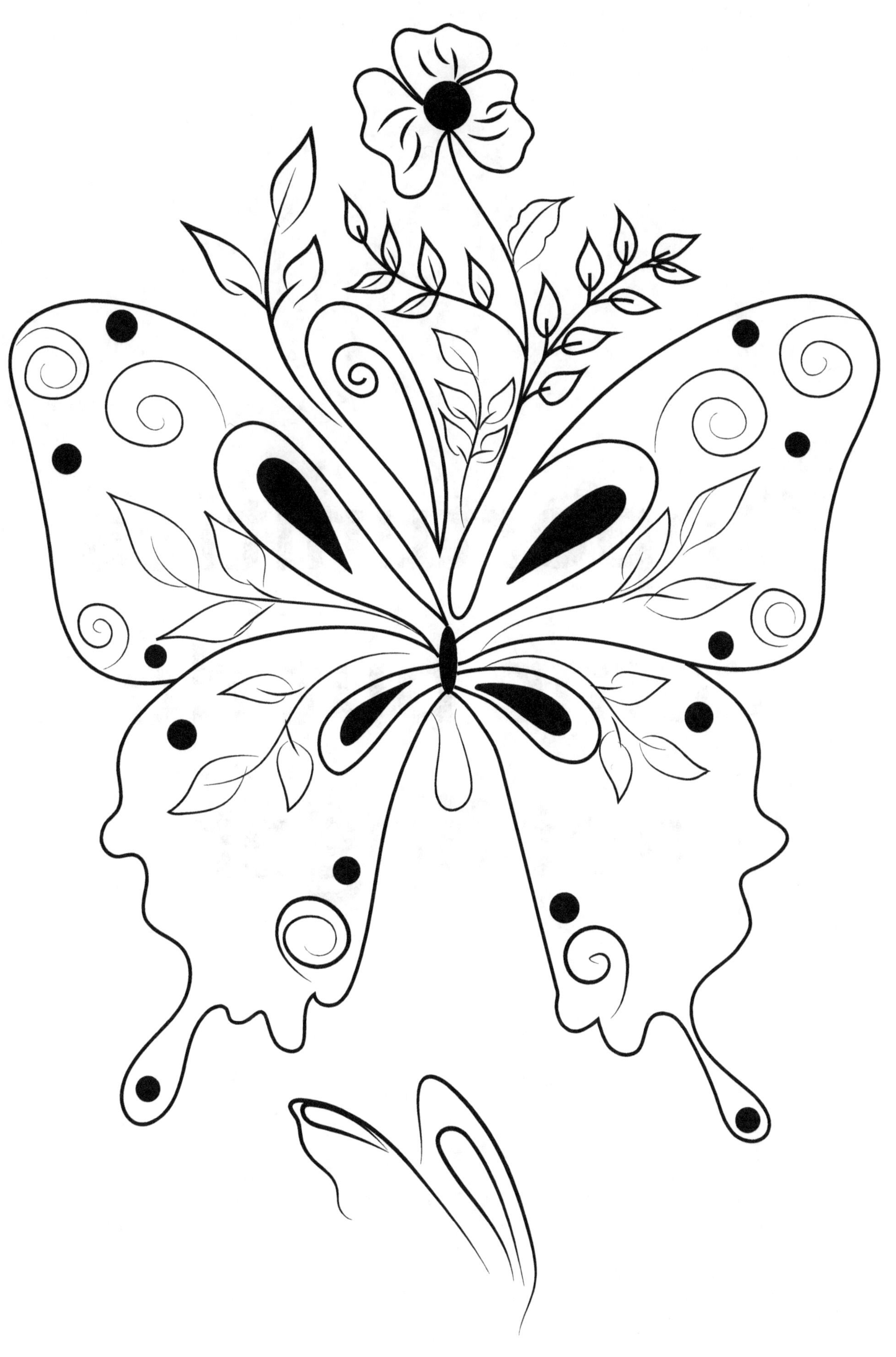

Opportunities come but do not linger

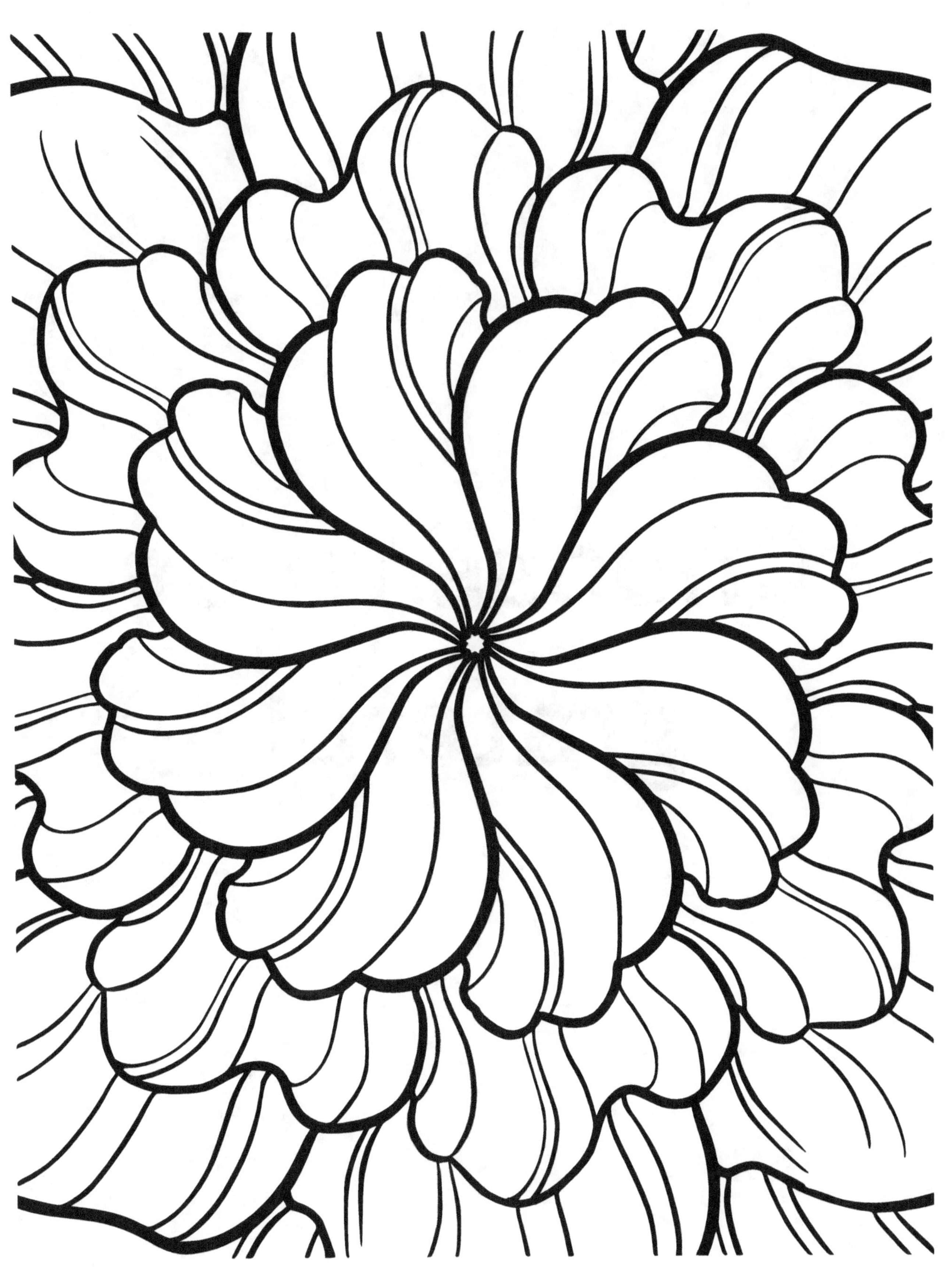

Choose to be grateful

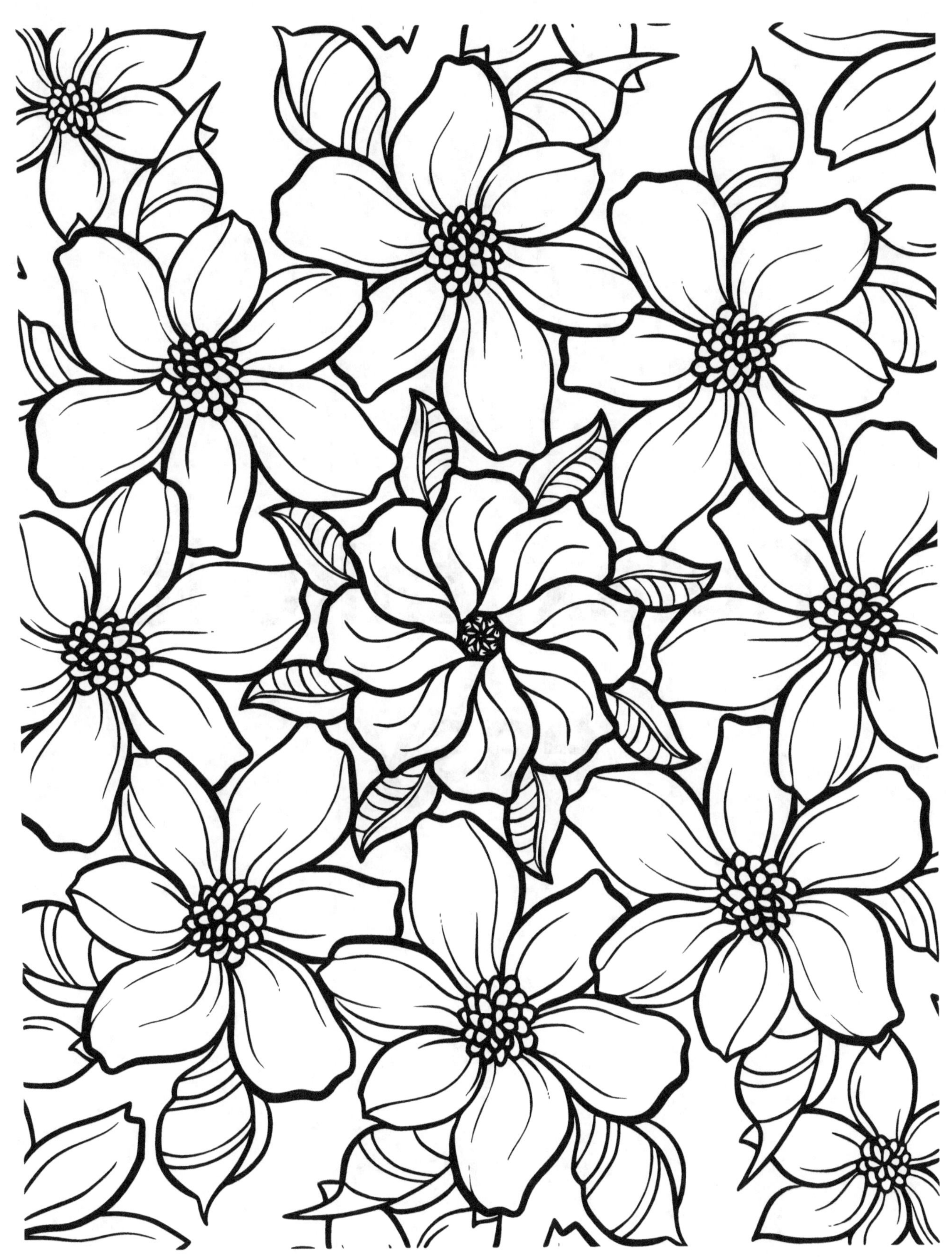

Relax, take it easy

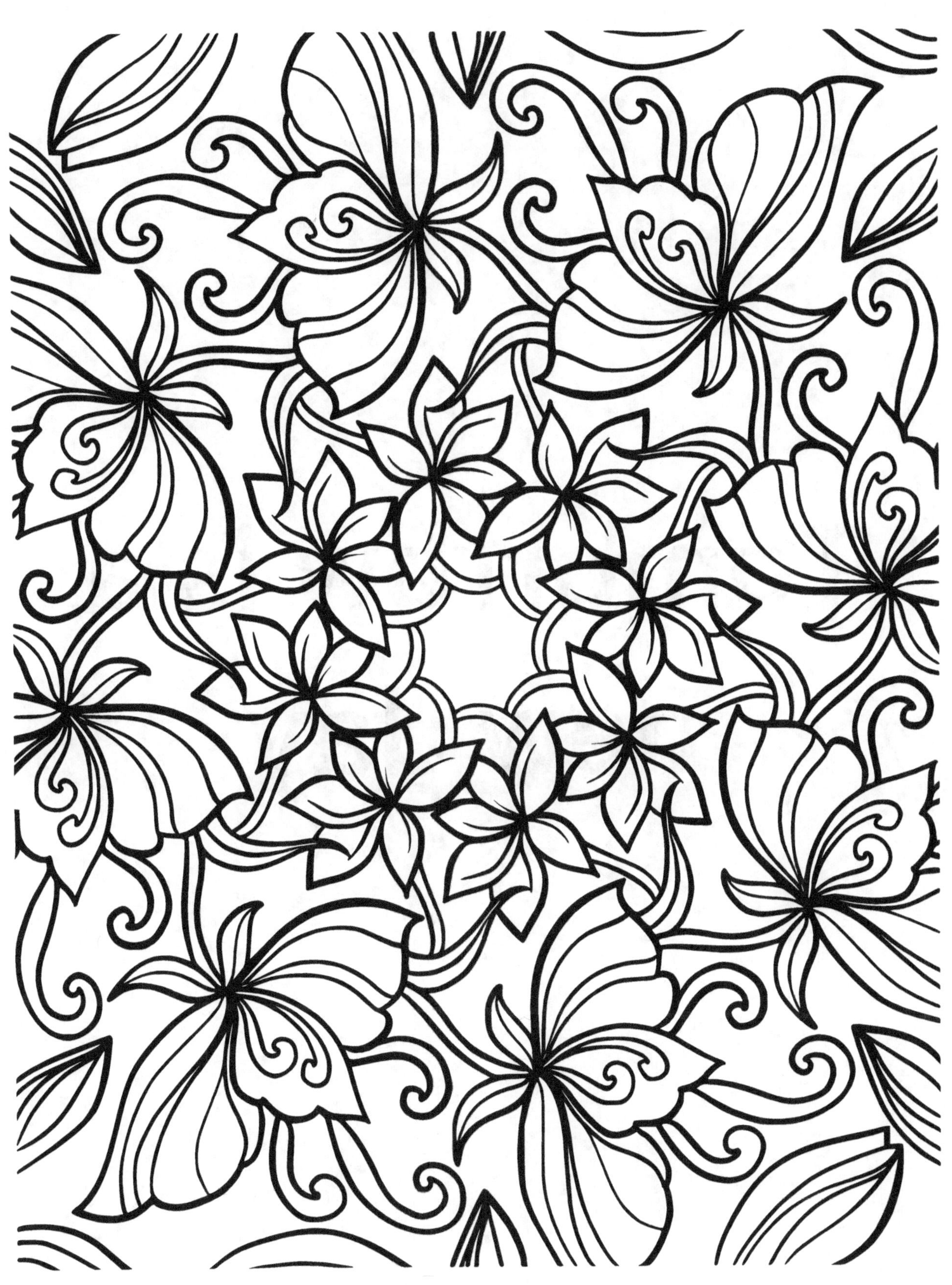

Tomorrow is a
new day

Make yourself
a priority

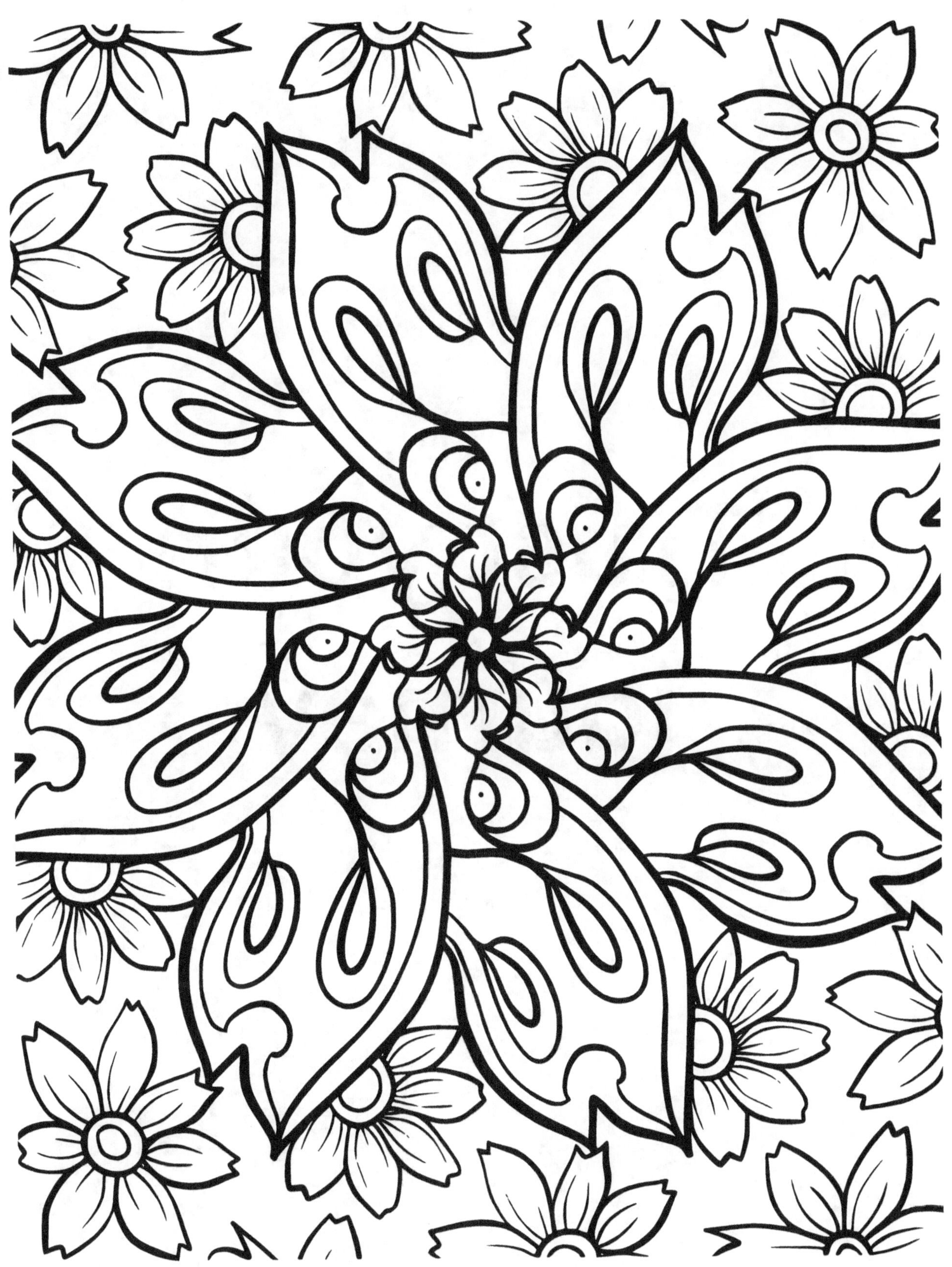

Trust your journey

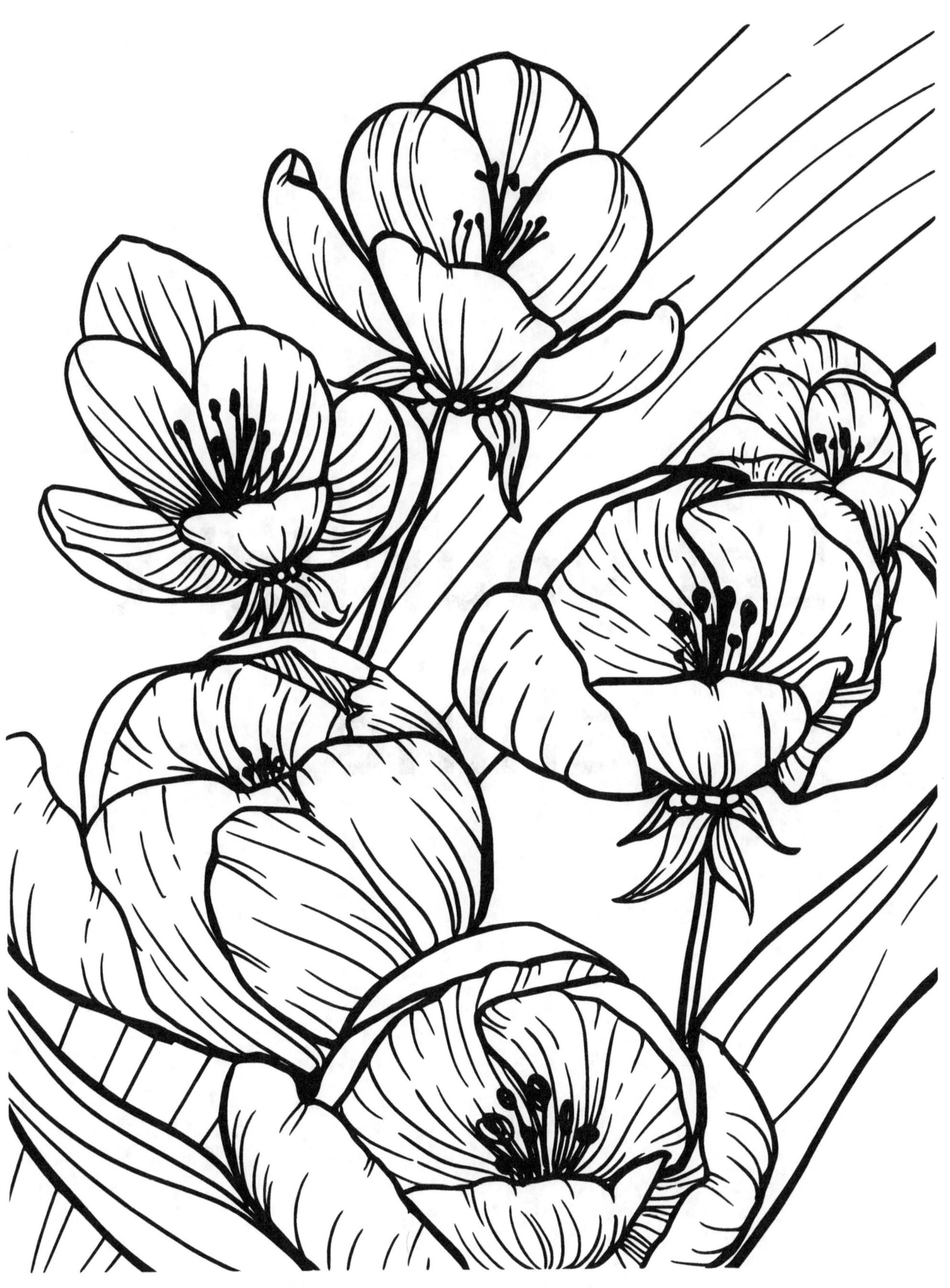

Let your light shine

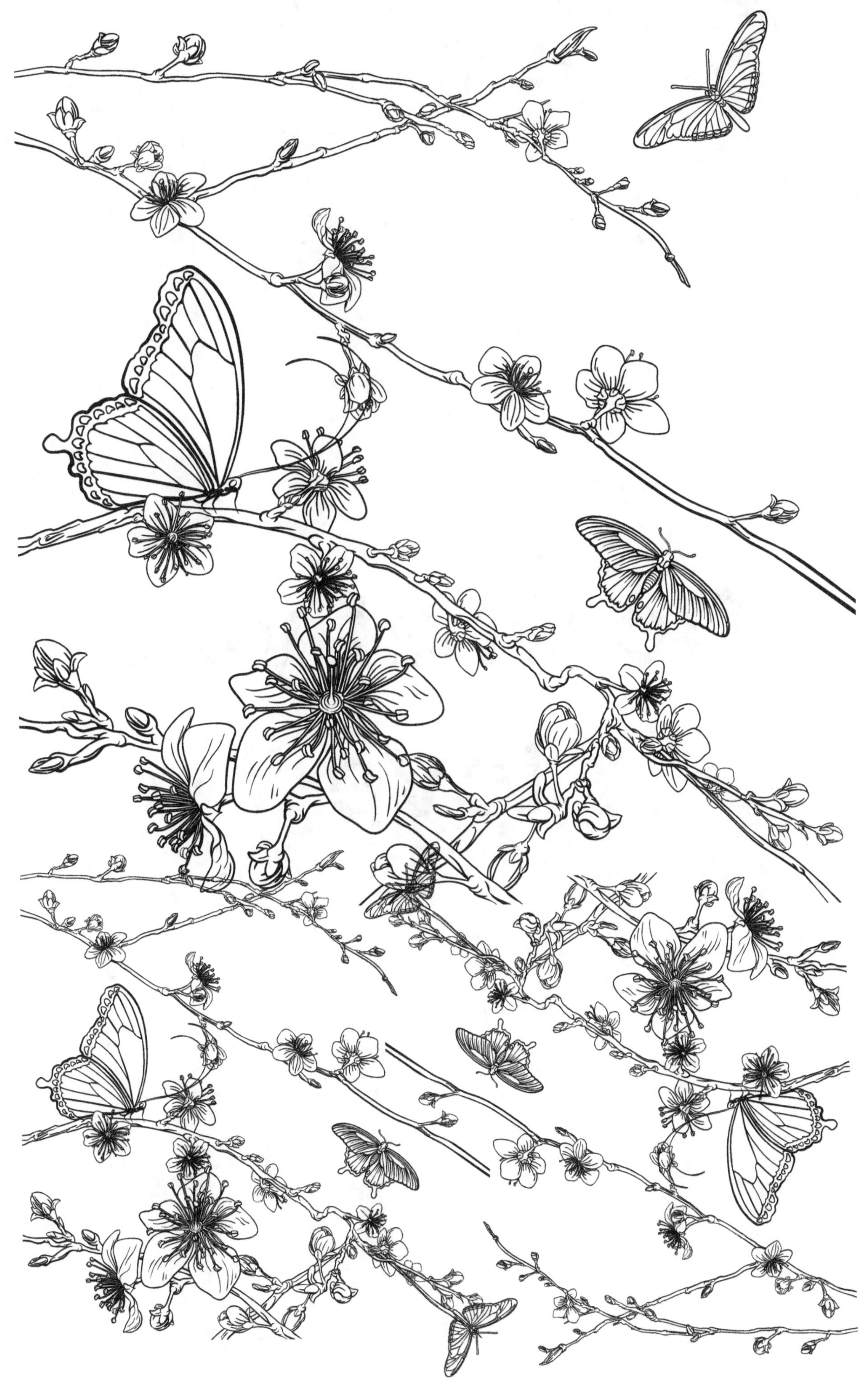

Do what you
love

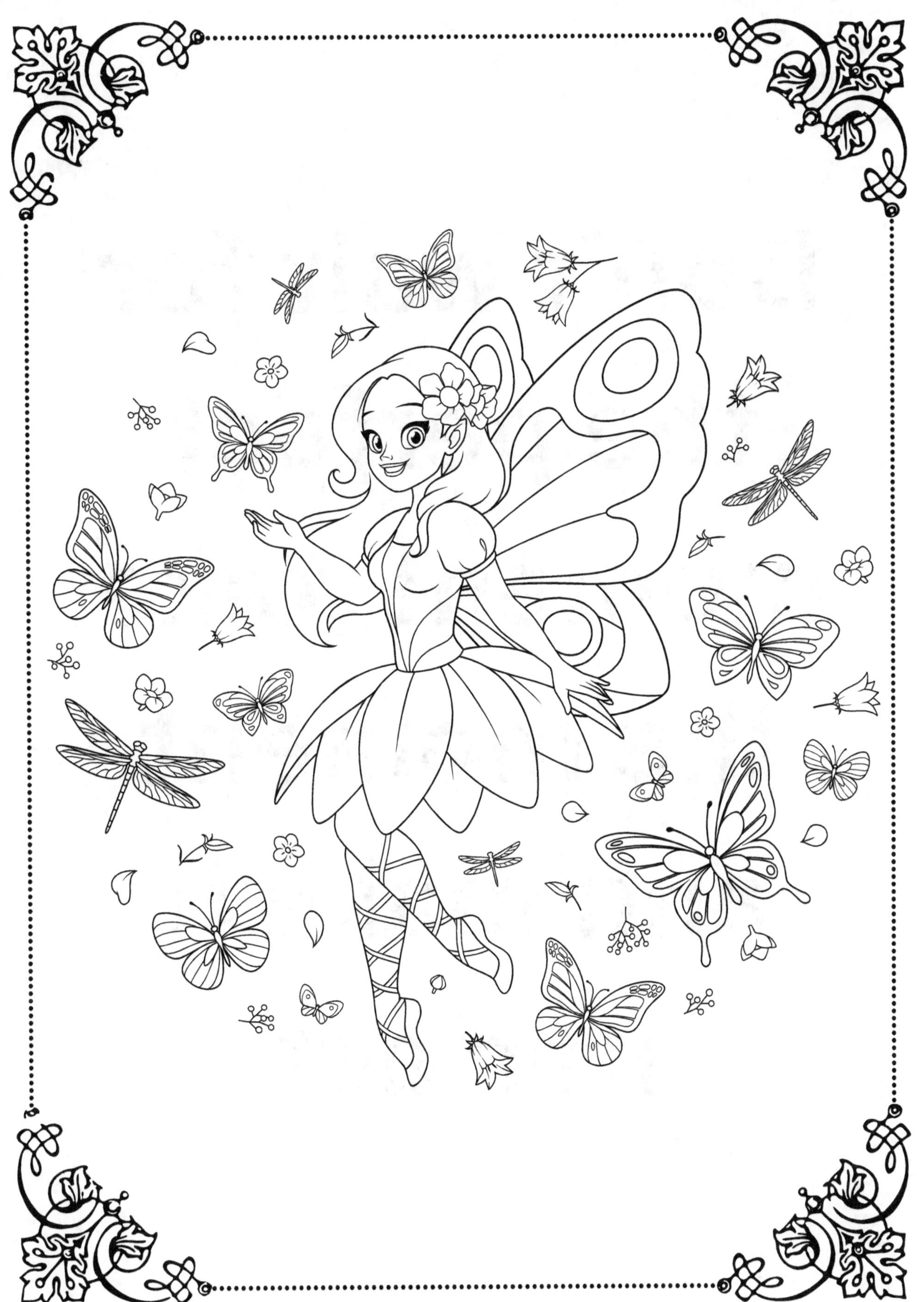

Don't wait for the perfect moment, take the moment and make it perfect